Healthy Eating for Life to Prevent and Treat Cancer

PHYSICIANS COMMITTEE FOR RESPONSIBLE MEDICINE

John Wiley & Sons, Inc.

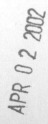

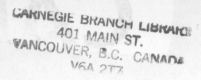
This book is printed on acid-free paper. ∞

Menus and recipes by Jennifer Raymond

Published by John Wiley & Sons, Inc., New York
Published simultaneously in Canada

Design and production by Navta Associates, Inc.

This publication is designed to provide accurate and authoritative information in regard to the subject matter covered. It is sold with the understanding that the publisher is not engaged in rendering professional services. If professional advice or other expert assistance is required, the services of a competent professional person should be sought.

Library of Congress Cataloging-in-Publication Data:

Healthy eating for life to prevent and treat cancer / Physicians Committee for
Responsible Medicine.
    p. cm.
  Includes bibliographical references and index.
  ISBN 0-471-43597-X (pbk. : alk paper)
    1. Cancer—Diet therapy—Recipes. 2. Vegetarian cookery. I. Physicians Committee for
Responsible Medicine.

RC271.D52 H43 2001
616.99'40654—dc21   2001046859

Printed in the United States of America

10 9 8 7 6 5 4 3 2 1

Physicians Committee for
Responsible Medicine Expert Nutrition Panel

Healthy Eating for Life
to Prevent and Treat Cancer

Neal D. Barnard, M.D.

Patricia Bertron, R.D.

Suzanne Havala, M.S, R.D, L.D.N, F.A.D.A.

Jennifer Keller, R.D.

Gabrielle Turner-McGrievy, M.S., R.D.

Martin Root, Ph.D.

Amy Joy Lanou, Ph.D.

Kristine Kieswer

Brenda Davis

with Vesanto Melina, M.S., R.D.

Special thanks to those who contributed to specific chapters, and provided thoughtful reviews or suggestions: John Borders, Wilma Glover, Jenise Sidebotham, Lavida Bond, and Sandra Howard, who shared their personal experiences; Staci Schmidt of the Block Medical Center, Bhora Derry, R.N., cancer specialist Abby Bloch, Ph.D., Brenda Davis, R.D., William Harris, M.D., and Hal Gunn, M.D., of the Center for Integrated Healing.

Contents

PART II: Making It Work for You

PART III: Lifelong Health

List of Recipes

Foreword

Cancer has leapt from being a fairly rare disease just a few decades ago to what is now a condition of everyday life. Far too many of us find ourselves in doctors' offices, having frank and frightening discussions about what this diagnosis means, either for ourselves or our loved ones, and desperately trying to sort through difficult treatment choices.

However, that dismal scenario is rapidly transforming into a far more optimistic one as we take powerful new strategies into our hands that can prevent cancer or alter its course once it has been diagnosed. These new approaches come from researchers who have carefully studied people with cancer and those seemingly protected from it. They have examined individuals who, despite the diagnosis, have lived far longer than expected or even had complete remissions. In tearing apart their diets, meticulously going through what they ate and what they avoided, clues have emerged that have then been put to the test in confirmatory studies. While this line of research is still ongoing, we have already learned enough that, if people everywhere took full advantage of it, most cancers would never occur.

Surprising as that may sound, one research study after another has confirmed that genes are not the cause of most cancers. Rather, our eating habits, aided and abetted by our smoking and drinking habits, are far and away the strongest determinants of whether cancer will loom in our future. Changing your diet makes an enormous difference. Whatever your age or current state of health, it is time to take advantage of this fact.

Perhaps the most important discoveries are for people who have already been diagnosed with cancer. Researchers have found that healthy diets not only make cancer much less likely to begin; good nutrition also can help a person already diagnosed with cancer to beat the disease.

Let me ask you not to keep what you read here a secret. Please share this vital information with your loved ones. Even better, try the recipes that put the science of nutrition into practice. They will do more than prevent cancer. They are also designed to cut cholesterol, help you slim down or stay that way, and introduce you to a world of healthy eating.

I wish you the best of success and the very best of health.

Neal D. Barnard, M.D.
President, Physicians Committee
for Responsible Medicine

PART I

Essentials

1

New Power against Cancer

If you or a loved one is concerned about cancer, here's wonderful news for you. Your food choices can cut the likelihood that cancer will occur and inhibit its course if it does. In the not so distant past, scientists had only the vaguest understanding of how foods might be able to help. Today we have powerful tools for naturally building a strong defense, and they are affordable and effective. In recent years, scientific research has made it abundantly clear that diet and lifestyle are formidable allies in protecting us from cancer. Because this is so important to understand, we'll look in detail at how the power of food choices became known and how you can put them to work. Better still, the second half of this book will show you that your defense system against cancer can be built up by meals that are absolutely delicious.

How do we know that diet makes a difference? In hundreds of research studies, scientists tracked how cancer rates differ among groups of people whose lives are similar except for the way they eat. In other words, their smoking habits are about the same, their genetic backgrounds are similar, but their diets are different. And by zeroing in on diet, we saw what happened to their cancer risk. Scientists set out to uncover this by comparing groups of people who are similar in every respect, except that one group eats more vegetables and fruits or more whole grains, or steers clear of meat and other fatty foods. In one study after another, the same pattern emerged: People who take advantage of certain protective nutrients and avoid risky foods have much lower cancer risk. If cancer *does* develop, these same dietary characteristics tend to improve survival.

We've heard that certain types of cancer, such as breast cancer, can "run in the family," suggesting that genetic factors are decisive and that diet may offer little benefit. But research shows that, although genetic factors do play a role in some cancers, the way we eat also "runs in the family." Food choices, handed down generation after generation, are a far bigger factor than our genes. A look at how cancer rates change as people emigrate from one part of the world to another is very telling. Their genetic makeup doesn't change, but dietary habits do, as people adapt to new ways of life. For example, when people moved from Japan to the United States, many traded their traditional diet, which had plenty of rice and vegetables and very little meat or dairy products, for a Western menu, heavy with meat and dairy products. With this transition, their breast cancer rates more than tripled, and prostate cancer became almost five times as common.

Cancer is currently the second leading cause of death in the developed world, and experts predict that it will not be long before it surpasses heart disease as our number one killer. Yet within this rising tide are strong indicators that we can prevent many cancers. When it strikes, we can influence its course to our benefit.

What Is Cancer All About?

Let us take a minute to understand what cancer is, to help us see how to tackle it. To many people it remains a bit mysterious—understandably so, because it starts deep within the cells of the body, complicated, minuscule structures you can't see with the naked eye.

Every cell in your body is an extremely busy little "factory," with thousands of biological and chemical interactions occurring every second. Each cell is working hard to control the use of oxygen and various nutrients, communicate messages, create new substances, and build new cells. In any given day, there are more of these regulatory interactions occurring within *one cell* than there are interactions among people in New York City.

At every moment of our lives, without our knowing it, the trillions of cells in our bodies avert potential damage and miscommunication, rid us of potentially toxic substances, repair injured cells, prevent cells with damaged genetic material from reproducing, and keep us in good health. Cells need the support of good nutrition to carry out this work.

Cancer begins when a cell goes haywire. As one cell divides into two in the normal growth process, it is easy for things to go wrong. In particular, it is easy for a cell's DNA—the genetic blueprint deep inside the cell's nucleus—to become damaged. If a cell is impaired so it begins multiplying out of control, that is the beginning of cancer.

Cancers most commonly occur where there is continual turnover and division of cells. For example:

- in the skin, lungs, and digestive tract, which continually slough off old cells and build new cells
- in organs that secrete substances, such as the breast, with its ability to produce milk
- in organs of reproduction: the uterus, ovary, and testes

In each of these parts of the body, cells are rapidly dividing. If DNA is damaged in the process, cell reproduction becomes disordered, resulting in uncontrolled cell growth. Eventually this growing mass of cells, called a tumor, invades the healthy tissue of the lungs, breast, prostate, or other part of the body.

How Cancer Starts

Why does the cell go haywire in the first place? More important, how do we hold cancer at arm's length (or farther)? Let's take a closer view of how this disease can develop and see where diet can intervene.

One way that food can affect cancer risk is by contributing carcinogens—that is, cancer-causing chemicals. They are found in tobacco, of course, and the same is true of some foods. Grilled, broiled, or fried meats contain heterocyclic amines, which form from certain compounds in the meat as it is cooked. Other troubling chemicals are N-nitroso compounds found in bacon, and aflatoxin found in moldy peanuts.

The trouble starts when a carcinogen manages to damage the DNA in one of your cells. The damaged cell can begin multiplying out of control. Uncontrolled cell growth leads to a clump of cancer cells, called a tumor, which can spread to nearby tissues or to the bloodstream, passing on to other organs in the body (metastasis). The word "cancer" is derived from the Latin word for crab and denotes a crablike growth that spreads throughout the body.

Powerful Protection Found in Simple Foods

The good news is that protective foods can enter the picture and change the story's outcome. They may block carcinogens from entering cells and reaching the DNA, or they can limit the damage that occurs. Even at later stages, out-of-control cell multiplication can be reduced or prevented.

For example, the mineral selenium found in whole grains and the brightly colored carotenoids found in vegetables and fruits have both shown the ability to slow, or even stop, cancer growth. Similarly, the vitamin folic acid, found in leafy greens, oranges, and legumes, also has been proven to protect DNA. Many other compounds have been shown to detoxify or eliminate substances before they can damage DNA, help defective cells return to normal, and put on the brakes before cells get out of control.

Does this mean we need to pile our breakfast table with endless vitamin and mineral supplements? Certainly not. The real magic is not in vitamin pills, but in eating the right foods. Foods are designed by nature to hold the protective nutrients we need in just the right balance.

These little brick walls show points of action for anticarcinogens.

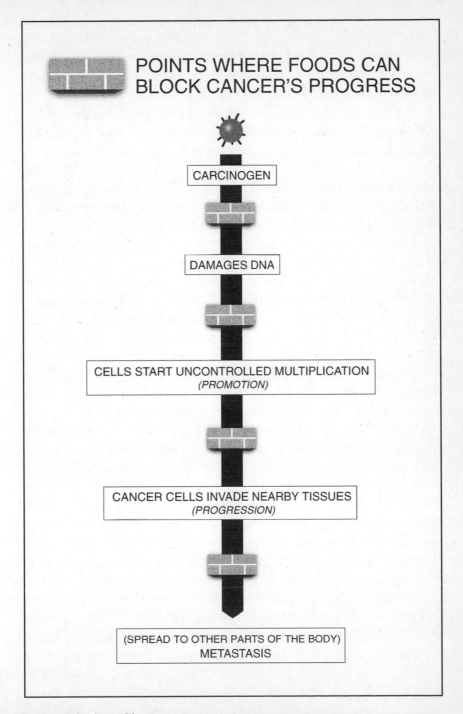

Cancer Blockers Chart (DOUG HALL © 2001 PCRM)

Cancer and Its Dietary Origins

While most of what we know about diet and cancer comes from recent research, the idea that foods play a crucial role in perpetrating and preventing disease has quite a long history. During the Song Dynasty in China (A.D. 960–1279), Yong-He Yan wrote that poor nutrition was a cause of esophageal cancer. In 1815 Dr. W. Lambe, a fellow of the Royal College of Physicians of London, wrote about diet, cancer, and chronic diseases, cautioning against excess consumption of food in general and meat in particular. His contemporary Dr. John Bell observed that some cancer patients had been cured by "adherence to a non-flesh dietary."

A hundred years later, Dr. W. Roger Williams noted, "Probably no single factor is more potent in determining the outbreak of cancer in the predisposed, than excessive feeding. Many indications point to the gluttonous consumption of proteins—especially meat—which is such a characteristic feature of the age as likely to be specially harmful in this respect." As contributing factors, Dr. Williams added "deficient exercise, and also lack of sufficient vegetable food." And Dr. J. H. Kellogg, a renowned surgeon who later championed the health value of breakfast cereals, echoed his views.

Despite the clear vision of these physicians, medical approaches related to diet and lifestyle received relatively little attention. Among mainstream cancer scientists, the search was on for something much more obscure than the food on our plates.

For decades during the middle of the twentieth century, most cancer research focused on specific cancer-causing agents such as radioactivity, chemicals in tobacco, viruses, and random genetic error as causes of this baffling disease. In time, more energy and increased research dollars were primarily devoted to *treatment* of existing disease—surgery, radiation, chemotherapy. In the flurry of activity aiming to improve treatments, prevention was neglected, and the role of foods was largely forgotten.

In the 1950s through the 1970s, textbooks that dealt with cancer's origins included little or no discussion of nutrition. Research hoped to find a single, identifiable, disease-causing substance or organism (as had been found with tuberculosis), and some magic bullet that could overcome it.

But cancer is not like tuberculosis or other infections, which arrive out of the blue and can be driven out simply by taking antibiotics. Cancer begins slowly, taking a long time to develop from a single cell into a noticeable mass. Its course is influenced by an immense number of complex, interactive events in our everyday lives.

Since the 1970s, scientists have begun to take renewed interest in the role of diet in causing cancer and in changing its course once it has begun. Looking at population groups with high and low rates of cancer, it became clear that cancer risk is not passed from person to person, like a cold or flu. Rather, the likelihood of developing cancer is closely linked to cultural tradition, especially our eating habits. Although heredity can be a factor, this is just one small part of the picture. After all, as we saw earlier, genes don't change as people migrate from one part of the world to another, or from rural areas to cities. Yet cancer rates do change, often dramatically, in direct relationship with changing food intakes. Here are examples:

- As Chinese people moved from Shanghai to the United States, switching from a diet that was primarily grain- and vegetable-based to a meat- and dairy-centered diet, prostate cancer rates increased up to fifteen times.
- Those who moved from Shanghai to Hong Kong and Singapore adopted dietary patterns that were midway between the plant-based and meat-based patterns. Again, rates of prostate cancer rose.
- When women moved from Japan to Hawaii and increased their intake of animal products, incidence of breast cancer tripled within one generation and continued to rise with the next generation, which had been raised from childhood on high-fat animal foods.
- In men and women who emigrated from Japan to Hawaii, cancers of the colon and rectum increased almost four times within one generation.

These migration and emigration studies provide compelling evidence that cancer is determined to a great extent by environmental factors, especially diet, rather than by genetics alone. Other studies, following large groups of people over many years, along with detailed comparisons of the diets of cancer patients and healthy individuals, established that diet is among the most important factors in cancer.

Today it is estimated that environmental factors, especially one's diet and smoking habits, bear primary responsibility for 70 to 90 percent of human deaths from cancer.

The Good News . . . Potential for Prevention

In 1997 a landmark document titled *Food, Nutrition, and the Prevention of Cancer: A Global Perspective* was released by the World Cancer Research Fund and the American Institute of Cancer Research. This 670-page report by an international panel of experts reviewed more than 4,500 scientific studies and summarized the effects of diet on the most common cancer sites. These are their findings:

LEADING CONTROLLABLE FACTORS ASSOCIATED WITH CANCER RISK

INCREASED CANCER RISK	DECREASED CANCER RISK
Smoking	Vegetable consumption
Alcohol use	Fruit consumption
Meat and dairy product consumption	Carotenoids (protective substances in orange, yellow, red, and green vegetables and fruits)
Animal fat/saturated fat	
Total fat	Vitamin C
Grilling and barbecuing (red meat, fish, chicken)	Fiber
Salt and salting (e.g., as a food preservative)	Whole grains
Obesity	Physical exercise
Inactivity	
Exposure to hazardous materials	

The message is clear. To reduce cancer risk, we can:

1. avoid those factors that increase cancer risk
2. bring protective foods into our diet and add moderate exercise to our daily routines

How powerful are these steps? Simply eating more vegetables and fruits could eliminate about 20 percent of cancers. By also avoiding animal products, we could easily double this number, preventing two of every five cancers. Regular exercise and maintenance of appropriate body weight can decrease cancer risk by approximately an additional 10 percent. Avoiding tobacco brings this figure up to roughly 70 percent. The remaining contributors to cancer risk include excess sun exposure; pollutants; occupational and environmental contaminants; and, to a much lesser extent, genetics.

Cancer in Various Parts of the World

Lung cancer, due mainly to widespread use of tobacco, is the most common cancer in the world. Beyond that, the situation varies immensely between developed and developing countries.

In North America, Europe, and Australia, hormone-related cancers (especially breast and prostate, but also colon and rectum) are most common. The meaty diets in these areas not only contribute carcinogens that can start the cancer process; as we'll see shortly, they also increase the production of hormones that can be a driving force behind these cancers. These fatty diets also promote obesity, increasing risk of uterine and breast cancers. Modern diets are also dangerously low in fiber (plant roughage), and the result is an alarmingly high rate of colon cancer.

For the next few decades, the picture for much of the world is not optimistic. With industrialization and the migration of people from farms and villages to cities, breast cancer rates are skyrocketing. Fast-food restaurants are springing up; high-fat meals, which allow greater absorption of carcinogens, are consumed at all ages; and the opportunity to grow one's own vegetables is becoming a thing of the past. Television, computers, and automobiles tend to keep us more sedentary than ever. As a result of these huge shifts in how we eat and live, our basic growth patterns have actually begun to change. Children grow faster. Puberty begins at a younger age:

5 years younger than it did 160 years ago. (World Health Organization records show that menarche, the onset of menstrual periods, in girls now occurs at age 12, compared with age 17 in 1840.) In turn, early puberty increases lifelong exposure to estrogen and a greater risk of breast cancer.

How can this dangerous trend be reversed? It's not likely that we'll all be heading back to rural living. But there's still a lot we can do about it. The following table shows dietary steps that can reduce cancer risk. They are easy, affordable, and effective. The percentage of cancers that are preventable are approximate and vary somewhat depending on the population under study.

STEPS FOR PREVENTING COMMON CANCERS

CANCER SITE	APPROXIMATE PERCENTAGE OF CASES PREVENTABLE BY DIET	EFFECTIVE STRATEGIES
Breast	33–50	High intake of vegetables and fruits Plant-based diet (avoidance of meat and dairy) Avoidance of obesity after menopause Maintenance of recommended weight Avoidance of alcohol
Uterine	25–50	Avoidance of obesity
Cervix	10–20	High intake of vegetables and fruits
Prostate	40	Avoidance of meat, meat fat, and dairy High intake of vegetables and fruits
Lung (for smokers and nonsmokers)	20–33	High intake of vegetables and fruits

Colorectal	10–20	High intake of vegetables
		Avoidance of meat
		Avoidance of alcohol

People in developing countries have some advantages. They are likely to eat less of the damaging animal products that are linked with cancer, and have lower-fat diets overall. But they do have problems of their own. Tobacco use is high. Protective vegetables and fruits are often costly and beyond reach. Many people have lost their land and their food cultivation skills, or simply moved to cities. Little refrigeration for perishable vegetables and fruits is available, and the use of high amounts of salt as a preservative has driven up certain cancers. While overall cancer rates are still lower than in Western countries, and hormone-related and colorectal cancers are rare, cancers of the upper digestive tract (mouth, pharynx, larynx, esophagus, stomach) and liver are much more common, reflecting use of tobacco and alcohol and a lack of consumption of protective fruits and vegetables. And, as people become more Westernized and adopt meat- and dairy-centered diets, patterns of disease begin to resemble those of developed countries. For example, cancers of the breast, prostate, ovary, and colon approximately doubled in Singapore from 1970 to 1990, as the country's dietary habits changed.

What to Eat, What Not to Eat

Combining immense amounts of data, collected from thousands of studies and millions of participants, the evidence is surprisingly straightforward. Plant foods and their protective nutrients reduce cancer risk. Alcohol and foods of animal origin (meat, dairy products, and others) increase risk.

The introduction of a wholesome diet, exercise, and other lifestyle practices at any time from childhood to old age will help promote health and reduce cancer risk. The same actions will help treat and prevent recurrence of cancer and cut risk of other chronic diseases. In the following chapters we'll focus on foods you'll want to avoid and those you'll want to be sure to include in your daily routine as strong allies for health.

2

Tracking Down
the Culprits

After researchers found that most cases of lung cancer could be traced to a single factor—tobacco—they trained their sights on other forms of the disease. And what they found has been disconcerting, because it is an indictment of some of the foods many of us have used as staples. But in the process, they have given us some vitally important lessons. In this chapter we'll explore how fatty foods, animal products, and alcohol encourage the progression of cancer.

What's for breakfast? Bacon and eggs, for too many of us. What's for dinner? Fried chicken or roast beef. In many families, fresh fruit, juice, broccoli, spinach, potatoes, and other healthy plant foods are not front and center, or may not even be part of the family meal at all.

Until about a century ago, much of humanity was suffering from a very different dietary problem. For the urban poor of Western Europe, meals were often monotonous and limited. Many impoverished children were raised on a thin white gruel made from cooked grains. A similar situation prevails in poorer parts of the world today. The science of nutrition, which emerged during the first half of the twentieth century, has been preoccupied with overcoming dietary deficiencies, and especially with getting enough protein. From this viewpoint, meat and dairy products were highly prized. They certainly do contain protein. But they also pack of load of fat, cholesterol, and calories, and are deficient in the nutrients that protect against cancer—vitamin C and fiber, among others.

Out of the Frying Pan, into the Fire

Skyrocketing obesity is a direct result of the popularity of burgers, cheese pizza, and fried chicken served everywhere. Hundreds of scientific studies connect animal fat with heart disease, diabetes, and cancers of the lung, colon, rectum, breast, endometrium, and prostate.

Fortunately, there are plenty of ways to get abundant, top-quality protein without these disadvantages. A varied diet of whole grains, vegetables, fruits, and legumes packs more than enough protein. And instead of being accompanied by cholesterol and loads of saturated fat, it comes with the nutrients that cloak your cells with protection against cancer.

Studies on thirty-four thousand American Seventh-Day Adventists, conducted over several decades, compared cancer rates of vegetarians and meat-eaters. Other aspects of lifestyle were similar; there was little smoking or use of alcohol in either group. Yet those who avoided meat, fish, and poultry had dramatically lower rates of prostate, ovarian, and colon cancer compared to meat-eaters. Even occasional meat consumption, red or white, increased the risk of colon cancer.

A twelve-year British study looked at cancer rates among six thousand vegetarians. It found cancer rates to be 40 percent lower than for nonvegetarians who were similar in body weight, social class, and smoking patterns—a powerful example of what a diet change can do.

Similarly, research in Germany conducted over a period of eleven years on more than eight hundred vegetarian men found cancer rates that were less than half those of the general public. Those who had avoided meat for twenty years or more had the lowest rates of all. Studies in Japan and Sweden also have shown lower cancer risk among vegetarians.

These studies have aroused great interest among scientists. How does eliminating meat lower the risk of cancer? If dairy products and eggs are also avoided, could this further decrease cancer rates? Over the next pages we'll see what scientists have discovered, beginning with some surprising problems of meat.

What's the Matter with Meat?

With every bite of meat you take, whether chicken, beef, turkey, or fish, you're getting more fat than you'll ever need or want. These highly saturated animal fats wreak havoc from head to toe, adding weight, disrupting your hormones, and escorting carcinogens into your body. And if you thought that cooking helped, there are more frightening surprises in store: heating meat unleashes a whole new batch of cancer-promoting substances.

Fat, Fat, and More Fat

The next time you think of animal products, think fat and cholesterol. To see why, look at the following table. As you'll see, both animal products and plant foods provide plenty of protein. The difference is that, in plant foods, the protein comes with much less fat and no cholesterol at all—the combination you're looking for in a cancer-prevention diet.

Fat and Hormones

The worst feature of the load of fat in meats may not be its ability to raise your cholesterol. It also increases the amount of certain hormones in your bloodstream—hormones that are linked to cancer. Let's take a minute to understand how this works, starting with breast cancer.

Estrogens are normal and essential hormones for both women and men. However, when there is too much estrogen in your blood, it can drive the rampant cell division that occurs in cancer. Many breast cancers are fueled by estrogen. And this is where diet plays a key role: the amount of estrogen in your body is linked to the amount of fat in your diet. If your diet is high in animal products and other fatty foods, your estrogen level is likely to be higher, too.

ANIMAL PRODUCTS VS. PLANT FOODS: NO CONTEST

ANIMAL PRODUCT	PROTEIN (GRAMS)	FAT (GRAMS)	CHOLESTEROL (MILLIGRAMS)
Beef patty, raw, 3 oz.	15	20	67
Chicken breast, raw, 3 oz.	18	8	54
Salmon, raw, 3 oz.	17	5–9	57
Milk, whole, 1 cup	8	8	35
Milk, 2%, 1 cup	8	5	18
Cheese, medium cheddar, 2 oz.	14	18	61
Egg, large, 1	6	5	212

PLANT FOOD	PROTEIN (GRAMS)	FAT (GRAMS)	CHOLESTEROL (MILLIGRAMS)
Lentils or split peas	18	0.8	0
Kidney beans, cooked, 1 cup	16	0.2	0
Tofu, raw, 4 oz.	18	10	0
Soy milk, 1 cup	6–8	2–3	0
Veggieburger*, uncooked, 3 oz.	17–18	0–2	0
Vegetarian ground "beef*," raw, 3 oz.	18–19	0.2	0
Vegetarian "chicken*," 3 oz.	17	2–3	0

* Brands surveyed were Yves, Nature's Chef, Field Roast, Lightlife, and Certified Organic.

When you adopt a plant-based diet that is lower in fat, your estrogen is likely to come down to a safe level, where cancer cells are less likely to grow. Most people are not aware of it, but it's vitally important for cancer prevention: when there is too much fat in your diet—whether from chicken, fish, burgers, or cooking oils—estrogen levels tend to rise.

There is also an important role for fiber in keeping hormones in check. Fiber—the plant roughage in greens, fruits, whole grains, and beans—actually helps the body eliminate excess hormones, cutting cancer risk: Here's how. Your liver filters your bloodstream. As blood passes through the liver tissue, hormones are removed and sent through a small tube, called the bile duct, into the intestinal tract, where fiber attaches to them, carrying them away with the wastes. Estrogen, testosterone, and even cholesterol take this same path out of the body—from the blood, through the liver, into the intestine, and out with the wastes. If you have plenty of vegetables, fruits, beans, and whole grains (i.e., brown bread instead of white bread, and brown rice instead of white rice), you'll have plenty of fiber to keep your intestinal tract healthy, to prevent constipation, and, perhaps most important of all, to keep this hormone-elimination system working properly. But if your breakfast was bacon and eggs and your lunch was yogurt and chicken breast, you have had no fiber at all. Animal products do not contain plant roughage. Fiber is found only in plants. If there is little fiber in your digestive tract, your waste hormones have nothing to attach to. They end up passing back into your bloodstream, circulating around and around, keeping your cancer risk higher than it should be.

Your liver is usually very efficient at taking excess estrogen from the blood, sending it down the bile duct and into the intestines, where fiber-rich foods carry it safely away. But typical Western diets are high in fat and low in fiber, causing estrogens to rise too high, overloading this effective system and allowing the estrogens to be reabsorbed in your bloodstream.

The healthiest diets avoid animal products completely. You've probably noticed more and more grocery store items labeled *vegan*—that is, pure vegetarian—as well as expanding vegetarian and vegan menu items in many popular restaurants. Diets rich in vegetables and fruits are naturally low in fat and high in fiber, and keep estrogen levels in bounds. These diets have an extra advantage. They increase the number of special "carrier molecules" in the bloodstream that pick up and harness estrogen molecules until they are needed. The result is fewer stray estrogens around to do mischief.

Fats in the diet begin affecting our hormones very early in life. A look back at not-so-distant history reveals that, in the mid-1800s, most young girls around the world reached puberty at about seventeen years of age, surprising as this may sound. In rural China, where low-fat rice and vegetable dishes are staple foods, this is still true. In America, on the other hand, girls are developing at age twelve or younger, and changing eating patterns are to blame. Chicken, beef, and endless fast-food meals are commonly eaten for breakfast, lunch, and dinner. High in fat and devoid of healthy fiber and nutrients, these meals are causing earlier puberty, and a host of other problems both physical and psychological. Most worrisome, they boost a young woman's lifetime exposure to estrogen, increasing her risk for developing breast cancer.

Excess fats in the diet are always troublesome, whether they come from plants or animals, and whether they are used in the kitchen or baked into store-bought items. But animal fats are especially harmful. Studies in the United States, France, Italy, and Sweden compared the diets of eleven hundred women with breast cancer to diets of women without cancer and found that those with cancer had been eating much more fat, particularly animal fat. Research conducted in Canada found that a high intake of animal fats doubles cancer risk. Similarly, studies in Argentina and Italy showed that high intakes of animal fats triple the likelihood of developing cancer. It seems that no matter what the genetic makeup, human bodies are hard pressed to withstand such a diet. Other hormone-related cancers—those of the uterus, ovary, and prostate—are also more likely with diets that are high in fat, especially animal fat, because estrogen and other hormones drive these cancers in similar ways.

Although men have a different balance of hormones—more testosterone and less estrogen—when it comes to diet, they benefit from exactly the same foods as women, making meal planning and eating out together that much easier and more enjoyable. Just as for women, when men eat fatty foods, their hormone levels rise. Male vegans, who eat no animal products, have plenty of hormones to meet their needs but manage to avoid the excesses. They also have more of the carriers that can hold on to excess hormones and prevent them from doing damage.

When a child starts out on a bad diet, its effects may begin very early, perhaps even before birth. One theory is that a boy's hormonal balance may be set very early in his development, leading to early puberty and high levels of testosterone later in life. Thus, if a boy's mother had a high-fat diet during pregnancy, the stage may be set for prostate cancer when he reaches his senior years. For now, this is simply a theory, and it certainly doesn't mean his fate is sealed. Most evidence suggests that the foods you choose even much later in life have a major effect on your cancer risk.

So far we have been looking at how foods can skew your natural hormonal balance. This is of great concern when it comes to cancers of the breast, ovary, uterus, and prostate. However, fatty foods also can increase colon cancer risk, albeit by a very different mechanism. Here's how it works. To digest and absorb a load of fat, your liver makes extra bile and sends it into the intestinal tract, where bacteria turn it into a cancer-promoting substance. But what really matters is not the biological details. What counts is what's on your plate. And the bottom line is that fatty, low-fiber foods pose cancer risks. Here are a few more findings you should know about.

Heterocyclic Amines

During the 1970s, Japanese researchers found that the surfaces of broiled or barbecued meat and fish contained potent carcinogens. These compounds, known as heterocyclic amines (HCAs), enter cells, where they damage DNA and start the cancer process. They form during the cooking process from creatine, amino acids, and sugars in meats, and all it takes is heat to turn them on. Roasting, baking, and deep-fat frying all create the same hazardous results. The higher the temperature and the longer the cooking process, the more these dangerous carcinogens form. Even concentrated meat juices, as in beef extract or bouillon cubes, may also contain these potentially damaging substances. Recent studies show that grilled chicken can be extraordinarily high in these carcinogens—fifteen times higher than roast beef or hamburger.

Some people seem to be particularly susceptible to these carcinogens because their bodies are slow to eliminate them. This may contribute to colon or breast cancer "running in the family." There is also evidence that heterocyclic amines may pass through breast milk and be transferred through the placenta to a fetus.

Grilled Meats and Polycyclic Aromatic Hydrocarbons

When fat from meat, fish, or chicken falls on the flames of your barbecue, polycyclic aromatic hydrocarbons (PAHs) are produced.

These carcinogens arise from the intense heat of a broiler or barbecue and are deposited on the surface of the meat, fish, or chicken. In their chemical makeup, PAHs are related to the cancer-causing substances in tobacco smoke. They can damage DNA and start the cancer process.

Cured and Smoked Meats

Nitrates, used in cured meats, form carcinogenic substances in our bodies. Two American studies and one Swedish study have linked use of bacon, sausage, smoked ham, and other cured and smoked meats with pancreatic cancer. These compounds may help start other cancers, too. Following consumer demand, nitrate levels are lower than they were twenty years ago, except in hot dogs, which still tend to have high levels. Luckily, veggie wieners are nitrate-free.

Pesticides in Animal Fat

Another disadvantage of animal products is that pesticides accumulate in their fatty tissues. While traces of these chemicals can be found on grains or other plants, when animals eat them, these traces build up in their bodies over the years. And if you then eat these fatty tissues, pesticides remain in your body for a long time.

Plant foods are generally much lower in pesticide residues, compared to animal products, and organic produce is lowest of all. The safest choice? A variety of plant foods that are grown organically.

Hormones

We've described how animal fats can disrupt hormone balance. However that's only one of the ways by which our hormone levels can be adversely affected by meat consumption. On North American farms, animals are given hormones to affect their growth: estrogens, testosterone, progesterone, Zeranol, and trenbalone acetate. A combination of estrogen and progesterone known as Synovex-S is sometimes implanted in the ear of steers. This is legal in the United States but not in Europe. The resulting estrogen levels in meat products range up to twenty times the levels in products from untreated animals.

Iron: A Double-Edged Sword

Iron is an essential nutrient required for healthy blood cells. But we need only a little in our diet because our bodies recycle it efficiently each time old cells break down. Too much iron is not only unnecessary, it also encourages the formation of cancer-causing free radicals, raising cancer risk. Studies at an American army hospital found that people with the highest serum ferritin level had a greater likelihood of developing the adenomas that precede colon cancer.

The iron in plants is in a form the body can easily regulate. It is more absorbable when you need more, and easier to keep out when you already have plenty in your blood. However, the iron in meat barges through your digestive tract wall and into your bloodstream whether you need it or not. If you were eating meat because you thought if was a "good source of iron," the fact is it may have given you way too much.

If you have any doubt, your doctor can tell with simple and inexpensive blood tests if you are meeting your iron requirements.

Red Meat, White Meat, and Even Eggs Are Trouble

When people try to improve their diets, their first step is often to reduce or eliminate red meat. That's a reasonable choice, but it does not go far enough. Though red meat and the fat it contains are heavily implicated in the development of cancer, animal products in general are hefty contributors. Whether it came from a cow, pig, chicken, turkey, lamb, or fish, meat harbors many substances that may support the growth of cancer. The Adventist Health Study showed that white meats add to cancer risk even when eaten only once a week. According to the researchers, these findings "suggest the presence of factors in all meats that contribute to colon carcinogenesis." As we've seen, grilled chicken is even higher than beef in its concentration of carcinogenic HCAs.

Like meat, eggs are high in fat and protein, but devoid of healthy complex carbohydrates and fiber. Considering their similarities in nutritional content, it comes as little surprise that meat and eggs may have similar effects. Evidence of this comes from the Adventist Health Study and from research done in Canada, Australia, Belgium, and Spain. An Argentinean study found that people eating just one and a half eggs per week had more than four times the risk

How to Check Your Iron Level

Your doctor or clinic can run the following tests. In some states, commercial laboratories will run these tests without a doctor's request. A physician should always interpret the results.

- Serum ferritin
- Serum iron
- Total iron-binding capacity (TIBC)

For ferritin, normal values are 12 to 200 mcg/l. Serum iron should be checked after an overnight fast. The serum iron measurement is divided by the TIBC, and the result should be 16 to 50 percent for women and 16 to 62 percent for men.

Results above these norms indicate excess iron. Results below these norms indicate too little iron. If the result suggests iron deficiency, your doctor may request an additional test called a red cell protoporhyrin test for confirmation. A result higher than 70 mcg/dl of red blood cells suggests insufficient iron. To diagnose iron deficiency, at least two of these three values (serum ferritin, serum iron/TBC, or red cell protoporhyrin) should be abnormal.

of colon cancer, compared to those who ate eggs less than once a month. You may not be eating scrambled eggs for breakfast each morning, but look at the ingredient labels on the breads, frozen foods, and snacks you consume. You may be eating more eggs each week than you ever imagined. A simple switch to healthier, vegan brands of common foods will put you on the right track. Eggs are the top contributor of cholesterol in our diets. Although we generally associate cholesterol with heart disease, dietary cholesterol has possible links to ovarian, lung, pancreatic, and colon cancers as well.

Dairy—Far from Perfect

The milk jug has long worn a halo in the eyes of Americans. However, in recent years the halo has become seriously tarnished. Dairy products have significant disadvantages when it comes to cancer risk.

Milk, whether from humans, cows, or other animals, is designed to help a baby grow rapidly. It contains hormones and nutrients that are tailor-made for the growth spurt between birth and weaning. But several of these hormones and chemicals also can give a real push to cell division and fuel the growth of cancer cells.

Insulin-like growth factor (IGF-1) encourages growth of the cells of the body. However, it also encourages cancer cells to grow and multiply. There are about 30 micrograms of IGF-1 per liter of cow's milk, depending on the stage of pregnancy of the dairy cow. The more milk you drink, the more IGF-1 ends up in your bloodstream—a major disadvantage, since people with high levels of IGF-1 have considerably higher risks of breast, prostate, lung, and colorectal cancers.

Exactly how milk increases IGF-1 in the blood is not clear. It may not be due to the IGF-1 in milk passing into your body. It is more likely that milk's load of protein and sugar cause your body to start making extra IGF-1 on its own. Whatever the mechanism, milk drinkers do seem to end up with more IGF-1 coursing through their veins, and this almost certainly puts them at higher cancer risk.

The Physicians Health Study in 2000 tracked 20,885 male doctors over 10 years, and it found that those who consumed 2½ servings of dairy products per day were 30 percent more likely to develop prostate cancer, compared with those using less than half a serving, and that includes both nonfat and full-fat dairy products. Similarly, the 1999 Health Professionals Follow-up Study, including 50,000 men, found that those who consumed the most dairy products had a 70 percent higher risk of prostate cancer. IGF-1 may not be the only culprit. Milk drinking causes several hormonal changes that would be expected to increase cancer risk, as we will see shortly.

Calcium, in excess, appears to increase the risk of some cancers, believe it or not. Milk certainly has plenty of it—about 300 milligrams per cup. Until recently, this was assumed to be an advantage. New research, however, has changed our view of calcium. First, while some calcium is needed in the diet, large studies show that people with high calcium intakes do not seem to gain any benefit for their bones, compared to those with more moderate intakes. In fact, in some large studies—notably the Nurses' Health Study in 1997 at Harvard University—milk drinkers actually broke more bones than people who generally avoid dairy.

More worrisome are studies showing that high calcium diets are associated with higher prostate cancer risk. At least sixteen research studies have shown exactly this link. Researchers now believe that high calcium intake alters hormonal balance, making cancer more likely in the prostate and possibly in other organs. Here's the problem: When you take in a large amount of calcium—from dairy products or any other source—your body reacts to the flood of calcium by reducing its activation of vitamin D (which is normally used by the body to increase calcium absorption). In other words, if you have plenty of calcium on board already, your body tries to avoid getting too much by reducing the amount of active vitamin D circulating in the blood. The danger in this situation is that vitamin D is also essential for keeping the prostate gland healthy. If there is less vitamin D in the blood, prostate cells have a tendency to become cancerous.

Ironically, milk is often supplemented with a form of vitamin D. But this form is biologically inactive, and the high calcium content of milk tends to prevent its activation. The moral of the story is this: To reduce the risk of prostate cancer, avoid dairy products.

Pesticides and industrial chemicals often dissolve in fat, and they can end up in mammary glands of cows and pass into your cheese, yogurt, and ice cream. Heptachlor, for example, was an insecticide sprayed on corn crops used for animal feed until 1983, when it was discovered to be a carcinogen. Not only did heptachlor end up in cow's milk, but also mothers who drank it passed it along in their breast milk.

Certainly it is a good thing that some dangerous pesticides and herbicides have been banned or severely restricted. Yet since heptachlor persists in soil, minuscule amounts of "unavoidable residues" are still permitted in milk, animal feed, and other agricultural products.

Estrogen, the female sex hormone, is also present in cow's milk in minute amounts. Part of the reason is that dairy cows are repeatedly impregnated until their usefulness is over. This is done because it stimulates mammary glands and supports maximum milk production. Pregnant cows produce extra estrogen that ends up in their milk. Excess estrogen is well known for making breast cancer cells multiply. This is why physicians avoid prescribing estrogen supplements to cancer patients. But don't wait for cancer to begin to bring your estrogen level down to a safer level.

Fat is a big part of most dairy products, including cheese, ice cream, milk, butter, and yogurt. About two-thirds of this fat is saturated fat, the kind that promotes heart disease. Though there has been a shift to lower-fat milks, American intakes of fatty cheeses tripled between 1970 and 2000. This fat adds to cancer risk.

As with other fatty foods, high-fat dairy products cause excess estrogen to be produced in a woman's body. As we've seen, high-fat diets have been linked to cancers of the breast, endometrium, prostate, lung, colon, and rectum. One way that fat may do its dirty work is by encouraging the absorption of carcinogens. For example, when carcinogens in cigarette smoke are absorbed through lung tissue, they travel along with fats in the blood to reach cells throughout the body.

A Little Douse Will Do You Harm

Though animal fats are a bigger problem than plant fats, substituting lots of vegetable oils isn't the solution. Polyunsaturated oils— corn, safflower, sunflower, and soybeans oils—can affect your hormone levels, just as animal fats can. They also contain unstable molecules that react easily with free radicals.

When vegetable shortenings emerged as "healthy" alternatives to animal fats, many people switched from lard to shortening for making piecrusts and other baked goods. Big debates took place about which was better (or worse)—the saturated fats and cholesterol of butter, or the hydrogenated fats of margarine. Don't debate about this any longer. Get rid of both. Cut way down on the fats in your diet, and build your menu from whole grains, vegetables, fruits, and bean dishes made without all those added fats.

You'll see how easy it is at the conclusion of this book.

Go Lean

One of the biggest problems with fatty foods, such as meat, dairy, and fried foods, is that they encourage weight gain. In turn, extra weight increases cancer risk. This is partly because fat tissue produces estrogens. In addition, many carcinogens are stored in fat (both the fats we eat and the fat on our bodies). These carcinogens come from air pollution, tobacco, smoke, other environmental contaminants, and foods. Happily, the same plant-based diet that offers so many other protections also helps trim your waistline.

Alcohol: Fuel on the Fire

Red wine made headlines about its possible benefits in relation to heart disease. Not to stop the party, but alcohol has no protective effect on cancer; in fact, the reverse is true. Alcohol is a carcinogen and a cancer promoter. It doesn't matter whether it's in the form of wine, beer, hard liquor, or a fizzy drink.

Alcohol is of greatest concern for breast cancer. The Nurses' Health Study showed that even one drink per day increases the risk of breast cancer. Just why this is so is not entirely clear. It does increase the amount of estrogen in the body, as has been shown in pre- and postmenopausal women. Alcohol also is able to affect the balance of insulin, estrogen, and IGF-1. Use of alcohol encourages cells to multiply and can hasten the development and spread of existing cancer.

When it comes into contact with the membranes lining the mouth and the esophagus, alcohol can ignite cancer here as well. In the upper and lower digestive tracts, alcohol plays another role as a cancer promoter, meaning that it encourages existing cancers to grow more rapidly. It also may enable carcinogens to pass into the mucous cells that line the digestive tract walls. The National Academy of Sciences, in its report on diet and health, does not recommend alcohol consumption. One of the easiest ways to lower your risk of cancer is to avoid alcohol.

The foods and beverages in your everyday diet have far more impact than most people suspect. Of course, cancer is not the result of eating one bad meal or a night of overindulgence. Instead, it reflects a series of choices made over many years. Luckily, we have many chances to tilt the scales in the right direction.

3

The Right Stuff:
Getting the Nutrients
You Need

Now that we are acquainted with both the foods that protect against cancer and those that promote it, the next step is to build an eating pattern to keep us healthy. Using the findings of cancer researchers, we can set some basic guidelines that will nourish every cell of our bodies with protective compounds. The energy that fuels our bodies comes from three essential nutrients: fat, protein, and carbohydrate. Achieving proper balance among these three has a great impact on overall health and risk of cancer.

Fat

With all you've read about excess fat disturbing your hormonal system and leading to obesity, you may wonder if fat is needed at all. In fact, we could not survive without it. Like shock absorbers, bits of fat cushion internal organs. A small amount of fat under the skin provides insulation from extremes of temperature. Fat helps us absorb vitamins, minerals, and the protective substances that assist us in fighting cancer. And tiny amounts of fat are used to build a great many substances that control our body processes.

Two specific fatty substances are needed. One is an omega-6 fatty acid (linoleic acid), the other an omega-3 fatty acid (alpha-linoleic acid). These technical-sounding names are not important. What does matter is that both types of fat are as necessary to life as vitamins. They form cell membranes, help substances pass in and out of cells, and are required for the brain, nervous system, and immune system to function properly.

They are not hard to find. They come from all sorts of plant foods, including some we may not associate with fats at all. For example, oatmeal, chickpeas, and leafy green salads contain a small amount of oil in every cell. Omega-6 fatty acids are present in all sorts of grains, vegetables, legumes, nuts, and seeds. Omega-3 fatty acids are less widely distributed. Our best sources of omega-3s are flaxseed, soybeans, tofu, walnuts, butternuts, and leafy greens. You may have heard that fish contain omega-3 fatty acids; however, the fish actually built their omega-3s from plants, too—from seaweeds and microalgae. In the Anticancer Food Guide on page 50–53, we'll list the best sources and exactly how much you need. As you'll see, it's not much.

People in Western countries often get far too much of the wrong kinds of fats. Animal fats and fried foods are everywhere. Sometimes manufacturers hide the actual amount of fat in packaged foods by listing only the fat content *by weight*. So whole milk, for example, is only 3.3 percent fat. But the fact is, milk is mostly water. Of the actual nutrients in milk, some is sugar, some is protein, and quite a lot is fat. So nutritionists prefer to list how much fat is in a food *as a percentage of its calories*. In this way, whole milk is actually 49 percent fat. In the same way, milk that is 2 percent fat by weight is actually about 35 percent fat as a percentage of its calories. In this book we will refer to fat as a percentage of calories, not as a percentage of weight.

Extra fat is not necessary, and it can do considerable harm. No one knows the precise amount of fat that is best, but good estimates range from 10 to 25 percent of your calories. You may have seen older guidelines suggest that 30 percent of our calories should come from fat. When reducing fat, don't stop there. Because fat intakes have been so high (34–38 percent of calories, and higher), 30 percent was suggested to give people an attainable, temporary goal. The World Health Organization, in its report called *Diet, Nutrition and the Prevention of Chronic Disease,* and the National Academy of Sciences have both advised that for health, the maximum amount fat in the diet could be dropped below 30 percent.

Protein

Apart from water, our cells (other than fat cells) are mostly made of protein. Protein helps our muscles contract and gives a framework to bones. Enzymes, hormones, and the molecules that act as messengers are all made from protein. Protein helps build the genetic material in cells and the antibodies that fight off bacteria.

The protein in our bodies is in a constant state of flux. Some of your cells, for example, may break down protein to its basic building blocks, the amino acids. These amino acids can then be used to build protein somewhere else.

Some people have the misconception that the more protein a person consumes, the healthier he or she will be. This is not true. As with fat, it's important to meet our needs. But beyond that, excess protein becomes a disadvantage. It puts stress on the liver and kidneys and is linked with other health problems, such as calcium loss.

For basic daily maintenance, nutrition authorities typically recommend about 0.8 gram of protein for each kilogram of body weight for adults, which works out to about 1 gram of protein for every 3 pounds you weigh. If you weigh 120 pounds, that works out to about 40 grams of protein each day. If you weigh 150 pounds, that's about 50 grams of protein, and so on. During times of growth or healing, a bit more may be required. Extra protein is required after surgery, radiation, or chemotherapy. This may increase your body's protein needs by 20 to 50 percent. However, note that most North Americans already get more than twice the protein they need, so there is not necessarily a need to add more. Some of the menus on pages 147–150 each provide 60 grams of protein. This is more than enough to meet the needs of an average adult.

The amino acids your body uses to build proteins are present in vegetables, beans, and grains. In fact, plants are the source of all essential amino acids—for people and for animals. You do not need animal protein, and are better off without it, because diets high in animal protein are related to increased cancer risk and are accompanied by fat and cholesterol. Plant protein comes with protective substances and without the damaging ingredients of animal products.

Many different plant foods provide protein. When your diet consists of a variety of whole foods, you'll get the most healthful sources.

Carbohydrate

The ideal fuel for our bodies is carbohydrate. In fact, our brains and nervous systems depend on it. Carbohydrate comes from the sun's energy, which is captured by plants through the process of photosynthesis and packaged into various plant foods. It takes the form of long chains of natural sugar bundled together with fiber. When you eat and digest these foods, their sugars gradually come apart and provide a slow-release energy source. Our systems function best when 55 to 75 percent of our calories come from carbohydrate. When carbohydrate intake falls below 55 percent, our diets are too high in protein and fat and there is greater risk of cancer, heart disease, and other chronic diseases.

Here's an important point about carbohydrate that many people don't understand. Carbohydrate is a real "Dr. Jekyll and Mr. Hyde." It has two faces, nasty and nice. The healthy form is complex carbohydrate, found in whole plant foods. Complex carbohydrate has that name because it is a complex mixture of natural sugars joined together, along with fiber and many protective plant substances. Healthy examples include brown rice, old-fashioned oatmeal, and the starchy parts of beans or vegetables. In contrast, refined starches have had their fiber removed and are left with few other nutrients. White bread and table sugar, for example, are refined carbohydrates that lack the goodness of whole foods. These refined foods send your blood sugar on a roller coaster ride instead of keeping it level, in the way whole plant foods do.

Some people say they feel a whole lot better when they cut down on "carbohydrate." The *real* story is that they feel better when they

cut down on refined starchy foods and sweets. They avoid croissants, French bread, sweet desserts, and sugar in their coffee. No
wonder they feel better. If people were to replace highly refined
foods with fresh-baked whole grain rolls, whole-wheat pita bread
and pasta, chickpeas and veggies at the salad bar, and lentil soup,
they wouldn't find that carbohydrates are a problem at all. In fact,
these healthy carbohydrates would be doing them a lot of good.

Fat, Protein, and Carbohydrate: Where Do We Find the Good Varieties?

When we combine the optimal amounts for the three major nutrients, we get a simple pattern: About 10 to 15 percent of calories
should come from protein, 15 to 25 percent from fat, and the
remainder—55 to 75 percent—from healthy carbohydrates. This is
ideal for healthy adults who wish to remain that way. During certain
phases of recovery from cancer, protein needs may be increased
slightly. Emphasizing some of the higher-protein foods such as
beans or lentils may be warranted at this time.

The following table shows the balance of these three energy-
giving nutrients in an assortment of foods. Beans, peas, and lentils
tend to be very low in fat. Soy is the exception, as it is a bit higher
in fat. That does not mean that soy is a problem, however. A review
of the evidence from dozens of studies shows soyfoods such as
tofu, tempeh, and soy milk either decrease or do not affect cancer
risk. Soyfoods contribute protective substances such as isoflavones,
antioxidants, and folate, and have top-quality protein. Food made
from isolated soy protein, such as some of the convenient veggie
"meats," can be very high in protein and low in fat. Products vary,
so check labels.

Soyfoods, nuts, and seeds can be valuable protein-builders and
energy foods during treatment for and recovery from cancer and are
far better for this purpose than animal products or refined oils. Any
of these can be added to blender drinks, stews, or casseroles, or
they can give creamy texture to a soup.

You may be surprised to learn that vegetables contribute protein. With a salad (two cups) at lunch and a sweet potato and a cup
of broccoli at supper, you'll get 10 grams of protein. For a woman,

who needs 50 grams of protein a day, this is 20 percent of her requirement just from vegetables alone.

Whole grains provide an ideal balance of protein and fats. For example, compare the figures for oatmeal, whole wheat bread, and the South American grain quinoa, to the recommended pattern for protein, carbohydrate, and fat given below.

PERCENT CALORIES FROM PROTEIN, CARBOHYDRATE, AND FAT IN PLANT FOODS

LEGUMES AND THEIR PRODUCTS	PROTEIN	CARBOHYDRATE	FAT
Black beans	26	70	4
Lentils	30	67	3
Garbanzo beans (chickpeas)	21	65	14
Pinto beans	24	73	3
Split peas	27	70	3
White beans	25	71	4
Tofu, firm	40	11	49
Tempeh	35	18	47
Soy milk	31	35	34
Soy-based veggieburger	56	28	16
Grain-based veggieburger	25	55	20
Vegetarian "ground round"	78	22	0
Vegetarian "chicken"	57	20	23
VEGETABLES			
Broccoli	34	57	9
Carrots	9	87	4
Cauliflower	26	59	15
Collards	27	65	8
Green beans	20	77	3
Kale	23	67	11

VEGETABLES *continued*	PROTEIN	CARBOHYDRATE	FAT
Potato	13	87	0
Romaine lettuce	36	54	10
Spinach	40	49	11
Turnips	12	85	3
Yams	5	94	1
GRAINS AND PRODUCTS			
Barley, pearled	7	90	3
Brown rice	9	86	5
Millet	12	80	8
Oatmeal	15	68	17
Quinoa	14	72	13
Wheat	15	80	5
Shredded wheat	11	85	4
Bran flakes	17	75	8
Pasta, white	14	82	4
Pasta, whole grain	16	80	4
Whole wheat bread	15	71	14
NUTS AND SEEDS			
Almonds	14	12	74
Cashews	11	15	74
Flaxseeds	17	25	58
Walnuts	9	8	84
FRUITS			
Apples	1	94	5
Bananas	3	97	0
Cantaloupes, melons	8	92	0
Oranges	8	91	1

Why Animal Products Are Not Recommended

In the following table, you can see the distribution of calories in some animal products. As you can see, fat is a prominent characteristic of these foods. There is no carbohydrate in animal products other than the lactose sugar in dairy products. In whole milk, half the calories come from fat; in sour cream, 85 percent.

Protein, Carbohydrate, and Fat in Animal Products, by Percent

Animal Product	Protein	Carbohydrate	Fat
Chicken breast	50	0	50
Salmon, Atlantic	52	0	48
Tuna, white	78	0	22
Beef, regular	25	0	75
Beef, extra lean	50	0	50
Egg	32	3	65
Milk, 2%	27	38	35
Cheddar cheese, medium	25	1	74

Foods for Health

This book will show you how to plan meals that will nourish and protect your body and, when necessary, help you to heal. Adapting to this way of eating may seem new and perhaps even a little daunting at first. But you'll soon see what a simple matter it can be. The recipes at the end this book offer excellent practical support for putting this guide into practice.

Strong Support for Plant Foods

Such a wealth of research has been done on the health benefits of vegetables, fruits, legumes, and grains that all major American health authorities have come out in support of diets emphasizing plant foods: the American Cancer Society, the American Heart Association, the American Dietetic Association, the American Academy of Pediatrics, the National Institutes of Health, the World Cancer Research Foundation, the American Institute for Cancer Research, and many others. These New Four Food Groups will help guard against cancer plus dozens of other benefits for your whole family.

Here are the keys to making the New Four Food Groups work optimally:

1. Build every meal from a variety of plant foods. Use fresh vegetables, fruits, legumes, and minimally processed starchy staple foods.
2. Eat *at least* five or more servings a day of vegetables and fruits, year-round.
3. Include legumes (beans, peas, and lentils) routinely in soups, burritos, as a side dish, or in new recipes that give delicious flavors to these protein powerpacks.
4. Eat six or more servings of bread, pasta, and cereal grains each day. Choose whole grain foods over more processed forms. Keep your intake of simple sugars to a minimum.
5. Limit consumption of fatty foods.

As you get used to your new routine, the following table may be a helpful quick reference to keep you on track, as well as a nice reminder of exactly which nutrients you'll get with each food you eat.

Ranges in servings allow for differences in body size, activity levels, and age. Smaller and less active people need fewer servings; larger, more active people need more.

By following this Anticancer Food Guide, your diet will provide a healthy balance of all essential nutrients. A few deserve special attention.

Calcium

Get to know better calcium sources within the legume, vegetable, and fruit groups. Calcium-fortified juices and soy milk are rich in

ANTICANCER FOOD GUIDE

FOOD GROUP: SERVINGS PER DAY	WHAT COUNTS AS A SERVING?	NUTRITION ADVANTAGE
Vegetables; minimum: 3 servings; eat these in abundance	½ cup vegetables 1 cup salad 1 cup vegetable juice	Vegetables provide vitamin C, beta-carotene, riboflavin, iron, calcium, and fiber. Orange and yellow vegetables are high in beta-carotene: carrots, red peppers, winter squash, sweet potatoes, pumpkins, and yams. Certain green vegetables (see calcium section) are particularly high in calcium, as well as providing these other nutrients.
Fruit; minimum: 2 servings	1 medium apple, banana, orange, pear ½ cup fruit ½ cup fruit juice ½ cup dried fruit	Fruits are rich in vitamin C, beta-carotene, and fiber. Include at least one serving daily from those high in vitamin C: citrus fruits, kiwis, strawberries, guavas, papayas, melons, and mangoes. Figs and calcium-fortified juices are good calcium sources. Choose whole fruit more often than juices, since fruit provides more fiber.
Legumes, nuts, and seeds; 4 or more servings	½ cup cooked legumes (beans, lentils, split peas) ¼ cup tofu or tempeh 1 serving veggie "meat" 1 cup fortified soy milk 2 tbsp nuts or seeds	Legumes—another name for beans, peas, and lentils—are excellent sources of protein, iron, zinc, B vitamins, and fiber. This group also includes chickpeas, baked and refried beans, fortified soy milk, tempeh, textured vegetable protein, and veggie "meats."

FOOD GROUP: SERVINGS PER DAY	WHAT COUNTS AS A SERVING?	NUTRITION ADVANTAGE
Legumes, nuts and seeds *continued*		Nuts and seeds also are part of this group. Of these, flaxseeds offer the greatest benefit, as valuable sources of omega-3 fatty acids (see below). Nuts and seeds provide vitamin E, selenium, fiber, and some protein. For most people it is best to limit nuts and seeds to one serving daily, due to the higher fat content.
Whole grains; 6 or more servings	½ cup cooked cereal, grains, or pasta 1 oz. ready-to-eat cereal 1 slice bread 1 oz. other grain products	This group includes breads, tortillas, pasta, hot and cold cereal, brown rice, millet, barley, bulgur, buckwheat, and quinoa. Build each of your meals around a hearty grain dish. Grains are rich in fiber and other complex carbohydrates, as well as protein, B vitamins, selenium, and zinc. Many are good sources of vitamin E. Choose whole grain products.

calcium, as are many brands of tofu. Most green vegetables are good sources of calcium: broccoli, collards, kale, mustard and turnip greens, chicory, bok choy, Chinese greens, and okra. Other sources are white beans, black beans, figs, almonds, and blackstrap molasses. To meet recommended daily intakes, have six to eight servings of these foods each day. This may sound like a lot, but it's as easy as having a cup of Cheerios with calcium-fortified soy milk for breakfast, baked sweet potato fries with a cup of white bean soup for lunch, and mixed vegetables (bok choy, kale, and broccoli are good choices) with marinated tofu over brown rice for dinner. Have a small handful of figs, almonds, or a glass of fortified orange juice and you'll easily surpass your recommended daily intake.

Vitamin D

Vitamin D is normally made in the body when sun shines on the skin. Ten to fifteen minutes of sunlight on the face and forearms daily are sufficient for light-skinned people; a little longer is needed for those with darker skin. People who live at northern latitudes or who do not get outdoors very often need a supplement or a breakfast cereal, soy milk, or rice milk that is fortified with vitamin D_2. Our needs increase as we get older. Following are the amounts to look for on supplement labels (in micrograms) or food labels (as the percent dietary value) for different ages:

	VITAMIN D_2	% DV
AGE	(IN MICROGRAMS)	(ON LABELS)
Adults up to 50 years	5	50
51–70 years	10	100
Over 70 years	15	150

VITAMIN D_2 FROM FORTIFIED FOODS OR SUPPLEMENTS

Vitamin B_{12}

Vitamin B_{12}-fortified foods and supplements are recommended for anyone whose diet is centered on plant foods. Many foods contain B_{12}, such as fortified breakfast cereals (Kellogg's Corn Flakes, Raisin Bran, or Total), fortified soy products, and Vegetarian Support Formula nutritional yeast. To be certain of a reliable vitamin B_{12} source, look for the word "cyanocobalamin" in the ingredient list. And, of course, you'll find vitamin B_{12} in any common multivitamin.

By the way, the need for B_{12} supplementation doesn't imply that plant foods are not nutritionally complete. Before such care was taken to bring immaculate produce to market, B_{12} (a form of bacteria) from the soil usually found its way to the table. These days you would find B_{12} in the meat of an animal who had ingested it, but the fat and cholesterol hardly make it worth the risk. Besides, the amount needed for good health is very tiny (2.4 mcg per day) and easily met.

Omega-3 Fatty Acids

To be sure you are getting the most healthful omega-3s in your diet, include one of the following daily: 1 tablespoonful of ground flaxseed, 1 teaspoonful of flaxseed oil, 4 teaspoonfuls of canola oil, or 3 tablespoonfuls of walnuts or butternuts. Ground flaxseed may be sprinkled on cereal, salads, or casseroles and mixed in blender drinks. Flaxseed oil may be used in dressings for salads, baked potatoes, vegetables, and grains (although not cooked or heated too high, as this causes it to lose potency). These two are the best sources of omega-3s.

Practical Pointers

Here are some pointers to round out your diet. Eat a wide variety of foods from each group: vegetables, fruits, whole grains, and legumes. Variety helps to ensure sufficient amounts of protective substances and also keeps meals interesting. Avoid concentrated fats, oils, and sugars, other than a small amount of flaxseed oil. These foods are high in calories but poor sources of nutrients. Get at least thirty minutes of physical activity each day. Physical activity, while not a component of "diet," is central to energy balance and to overall health. If you are over forty, or have any health concern, be sure to check with your doctor before you begin.

While nutrition research has been extraordinarily detailed and complex, planning your meals is easy. By focusing on vegetables, fruits, whole grains, and legumes, you'll be taking full advantage of the good nutrition nature has to offer.

PART II

Making It Work for You

4

Cancer:
Dietary Self-Defense

Our defense against cancer is built of simple choices we make at every meal. A colorful salad, a glass of carrot juice, a crusty whole-grain roll, tamale pie, a fruit crisp. A walk during your lunch break, breaths of fresh, clean air. These are the life-affirming choices that seem so simple on their own but that can cut your risk of cancer over the days, months, and years. In this chapter you'll learn why antioxidants in vegetables and fruits, fiber in whole grains and other foods, and other cancer-fighters, from herbs to soy, are such strong allies for health.

Plant foods are packed with protective compounds that guard our lungs from carcinogens in the air. For women, they protect breast tissue against the onslaught of too much estrogen. For men, they defend the prostate against hormones and harmful dietary components. The National Cancer Institute has recognized dozens of foods as having specific anticancer properties, and the list is growing constantly. Let's take a closer look at how they perform their everyday miracles.

Veggies, Fruits, and Natural Antioxidants

If the word "vegetables" doesn't conjure up in your mind sensations of color, fragrance, delicious flavor, and bountiful health, it's time to update your attitudes about these amazing foods. Forget the piece of overcooked broccoli you were reluctant to eat at age four. Turn your attention to spinach burritos, salsa, gazpacho, grilled Portobello mushroom "steaks," tomato soup, or an autumn vegetable stew. When you have a savory soup and salad for lunch, and build your dinner around veggies, you consume a host of protective vitamins, minerals, and other compounds. More than any other group of foods, vegetables have proven their worth as cancer fighters. This is a great time to make the acquaintance of some new members of this colorful family of plant foods, and see what friends they can be in supporting your health.

Fruits are nature's sweetest protection. The benefits of fruits against cancers of the lung, breast, prostate, colon, and other sites have been clearly shown. Like vegetables, they hold an abundance of antioxidants, a wealth of other anticancer compounds, and fiber.

The cancer-fighting power of vegetables and fruits comes in large part from their ability to knock out free radicals—unstable molecules that can spark the onset of cancer. Let's take a moment to understand how they work.

Vegetables or Fruits?

Q Are avocados, cucumbers, eggplants, peppers, pumpkins, squash, tomatoes, and zucchini fruits or vegetables?

A A fruit is the part of a plant involved in its reproduction; fruits contain seeds. So, although these foods are not sweet like an apple or an orange, botanically speaking, all are fruits. Other parts of plants are vegetables: the stems (asparagus, celery), roots (beet, carrot), flowers (broccoli, cauliflower), leaves (greens), and bulbs (garlic) or tubers (potato, sweet potatoes, yams) that grow underground. When it comes to cancer-fighting, it doesn't matter how they're classified. They *all* offer protection.

The Antioxidant Arsenal

Oxygen is fundamental to life. Yet, as our cells use oxygen for various purposes, some molecules of this essential substance can become very unstable, with the potential to wreak havoc in our bodies. If you could look at them through a powerful microscope, you would see that the chemical reactions in the body have left them with too many electrons, or electrons in unstable orbits. In this form, oxygen molecules are called free radicals. What is important is that these highly reactive molecules roam around the body looking for other molecules with which to react. When free radicals attack the molecules that make up your skin, the results are wrinkles and other signs of aging. When they attack the DNA inside your cells, however, the results can be that cells begin multiplying out of control, the start of cancer.

When our diets are out of balance, two big problems commonly arise. First, we may produce too many free radicals. For example, certain foods (such as meats that contribute nitrates) feed free radical formation, as do cigarette smoke and alcohol. Second, we may not eat enough antioxidant-rich plant foods to keep free radicals in check.

Although free radicals can easily start the cancer process by attacking your DNA, a diet with enough protective compounds can quickly halt the damage, stopping cancer in its tracks.

Antioxidants are the heroes that protect DNA against carcinogens. They put free radicals out of commission. Without continual antioxidant action, we would not survive. And without plenty of antioxidant-rich plant foods, we place tremendous pressure on our cells, some to the point of defeat. Antioxidants also help in the fight against existing cancer. They prevent further injury to DNA and other parts of cells. Four key antioxidants are vitamin C, beta-carotene, vitamin E, and selenium.

Vitamin C

Vitamin C is a great team player in the antioxidant defense system. It protects against free radical damage and keeps the linings of our lungs, stomach, and reproductive organs in good repair. In grade school we learned that orange juice is a potent source of vitamin C, but that's just the beginning. As you can see in the table on pages 50–53, we get this cancer-fighting vitamin from many vegetables such as yams, sweet potatoes, broccoli, and others in the cabbage family, such as kale. And, of course, it's also in a wide assortment of fruits.

To illustrate vitamin C's importance, let's look at lung cancer. Needless to say, smoking is a big part of the problem. Compared to a nonsmoker, a lifetime smoker has twenty to thirty times the risk of getting lung cancer. Secondhand smoke is dangerous, too, increasing lung cancer risk by 30 to 50 percent. But just as tobacco increases the risk of cancer, foods rich in vitamin C reduce the likelihood that lung cancer will start. In other words, you can protect the delicate linings of your lungs against pollutants with vitamin C–rich fruits and vegetables at every meal.

Both nonsmokers *and* smokers benefit from these foods. Let's compare two fifty-five-year-old smokers, Veggie Vic and Pretzel Pete. Vic's typical menu on any given day looks something like this: oatmeal with fresh berries, a slice of cantaloupe, and a cup of tea for breakfast, a banana and orange juice smoothie for a snack, a veggie sub on wheat bread and a bowl of minestrone for lunch, and hearty pasta with tomatoes, eggplant, and basil for dinner. With his preference for these healthy and delicious foods, Vic has just *one-quarter* the risk of dying from lung cancer during the next four years, compared with Pete, who munches on pretzels and other highly refined foods, hardly thinking of eating a vegetable or a fruit.

Beta-carotene

Beta-carotene is part of a family of more than six hundred different carotenoids. They give vibrant color to carrots, red peppers, sweet potatoes, yams, apricots, cantaloupes, mangoes, pumpkins, and many other foods with similar hues. Kale and spinach are rich in beta-carotene, too, although the green of chlorophyll hides its pale orange color. Beta-carotene knocks out free radicals and strengthens special white blood cells called natural killer cells, which seek out and destroy cancer cells.

How much of these protective foods do we need? With five servings a day of vegetables and fruits, you'll get a supply of about 800 to 1,000 micrograms of beta-carotene. You'll want to get at least this much each day. To see whether your diet meets this lower limit, jot down the vegetables and fruits you ate yesterday. Then look at the table on pages 50–53 and add up your intake of beta-carotene. It's smart to boost your intake even higher, to 30,000 micrograms or more of beta-carotene, by regularly including the richest sources in your diet.

Here are three different ways to get 30,000 micrograms of beta-carotene:

- two large carrots
- one cup of baked yam or sweet potato, one cup of kale, and a peach
- a wedge of cantaloupe, 8 ounces of carrot juice, plus a half cup of cooked pumpkin

Five a Day: The Minimum

Research has shown that a daily intake of five servings of vegetables and fruit would eliminate at least one in five cases of cancer, even if the rest of the diet was not changed at all. A typical serving means ½ cup of fruit or vegetables, a single medium-sized vegetable (carrot, apple, tomato), 1 cup of salad, or ¾ cup of juice. If your day's intake doesn't include five of these foods, here are examples to get you started.

Getting Enough Vegetables and Fruits?

The average American eats only two and a half servings daily, and that's counting the fries! Just one person in eleven consumes the five servings recommended by the National Cancer Institute. In fact, studies show that over the course of a day, almost half the population has no fruit or juice at all. One person in five has eaten no vegetables. No wonder cancer is so common.

Minimum Day's Intake for Vegetables and Fruit

Meal	Example 1	Example 2	Example 3	Example 4
Breakfast	Blueberries, ½ cup	Apple, 1	Grapefruit or orange juice, ¾ cup	Papaya, ½ cup
Lunch	Vegetable soup, ½ cup vegetables	Salad, 2 cups (counts as 2 servings)	Raw veggie strips: carrots, sweet red pepper, celery, 1 cup (counts as 2 servings)	Tomato sauce with onion, garlic, and mushrooms, 1 cup (counts as 2 servings)
Dinner	Yam, ½ cup Broccoli, ½ cup	Corn, ½ cup	Tomato, 1	Steamed kale, ½ cup
Snack	Fruit juice, ¾ cup	Orange, 1	Berries or seasonal fruit, ½ cup	Banana, 1

Higher intakes of vegetables and fruit are even more protective, so don't be shy. Although government food guides generally list ½ cup as a serving, pile your plate with double or triple that amount. These foods won't make you fat. What they *will* do is boost your intake of antioxidants, vitamins, and minerals. The recipe section and the menus in the back of the book show you how to build meals around vegetables and make delicious fruit-based desserts.

You may be thinking, "That may work when I'm home, but what about when I'm out?" Here are some tips. When you travel, and on social occasions, choose fruit juice. It's widely available from vending machines and even at fast-food outlets. Americans drink 597 cans of soda per person per year. Think of the increase in vitamin C if they switched to orange juice! Keep a bowl of fruit on the table, and pop some fruit into your bag as you head out the door. Cut up raw veggies, and keep a container of them in your refrigerator. Instead of splurging on junk food, try papayas, blue-berries, or red peppers.

Vitamin E

Vitamin E is a popular seller in the vitamin aisle, but let's not for-get where it comes from originally. Vitamin E is naturally present in plant oils. Its specialty is protecting cell membranes. The delicate membranes covering each of your cells are vulnerable to attack by free radicals, leaving you wide open to DNA damage. Vitamin E can stop that chain reaction in its tracks.

Vitamin E also supports your immune system, guards against heart disease, and may even protect against gallstones and cataracts. Where do we find this powerful vitamin? It's in green vegetables, orange-colored fruits, and blueberries. You'll get even more from whole grains, legumes, nuts, and seeds. Note that the natural form of vitamin E, present in all these foods, is more potent, more available, and lasts longer in the body, compared with the syn-thetic vitamin E in supplements.

Selenium

The fourth member of this antioxidant team is the mineral selenium. It is a silvery-colored mineral that was named for Selene, the ancient Greek goddess of the moon. It works together with vitamin E to protect cells against damage from free radicals and other carcino-gens. Studies done at Harvard and Cornell Universities and in China have shown selenium levels to be 30 to 40 percent lower in cancer patients than in healthy people. Low selenium levels have been linked to cancers of the digestive system and the prostate.

A surprising number of foods provide this powerful antioxidant. Take garlic as an example. A clove here and there adds up. When you learn to flavor recipes with garlic, you'll wonder why you ever used so much salt. Over the course of a day, a diet rich in vegetables and fruits provides some selenium, and you'll get even higher amounts from whole grains (barley, brown rice, oatmeal), legumes, seeds, and nuts. Mushrooms are good sources; tofu and Brazil nuts are excellent sources.

ANTIOXIDANTS IN FOODS

SERVING SIZE: 1 CUP, RAW, UNLESS SPECIFIED	VITAMIN, C, MG*	BETA-CAROTENE MCG[†]	VITAMIN E, MG	SELENIUM, MCG
Daily target, minimum	Women, 75; Men, 90	Women, 800; Men, 1,000	15	55
Vegetables				
Bell pepper, red	175	2,840	0.7	0.3
Broccoli	82	807	1.5	3
Brussels sprouts, cooked	97	669	1.3	2
Cabbage	29	69	1.5	1
Carrot, large (4 oz), 1	11	15,503	0.7	1
Carrot juice	20	12,559	1	1
Cauliflower	46	12	0.1	1
Garlic	42	0	0	19
Kale	80	3,577	0.5	1
Leeks, cooked	4	31	0.7	1
Mushrooms	2	0	0.3	8
Onions, white, cooked	11	0	0.8	1
Potato, medium, baked, 1	16	0	0.1	1
Pumpkin, cooked	10	31,908	2.6	1
Spinach	8	1,196	0.8	0.3
Squash, acorn, cooked	26	627	1.6	2

SERVING SIZE: 1 CUP, RAW, UNLESS SPECIFIED	VITAMIN, C, MG*	BETA-CAROTENE MCG†	VITAMIN E, MG	SELENIUM, MCG
Vegetables continued				
Sweet potato, cooked	49	26,184	0.6	1
Tomato, medium	23	446	1.1	0.5
Yam, orange, baked	49	26,184	0.6	1
Fruits				
Apple, medium	8	28	0.9	0.4
Apricots, 3	10	1,635	0.9	0.4
Banana, medium	11	57	0.4	1.3
Blueberries	19	87	2.7	1
Cantaloupe (⅛ melon)	29	1,325	0.2	0.3
Cantaloupe, cubes	68	3,072	0.5	0.6
Grapefruit sections	79	160	0.6	3
Grapes	4	54	0.3	0.2
Guava	303	750	1.8	1
Kiwi, 2	114	164	1.7	0.6
Mango	46	3,851	1.8	1
Orange, medium	59	52	0.4	1
Orange juice	124	92	0.5	0.2
Papaya	87	70	1.6	0.8
Peach	6	260	1	0.4
Raspberries	31	48	0.6	0.7
Strawberries	82	23	0.4	1
Watermelon, 1/16	27	634	0.4	0.3

SERVING SIZE: 1 CUP, RAW, UNLESS SPECIFIED	VITAMIN, C, MG*	BETA-CAROTENE MCG†	VITAMIN E, MG	SELENIUM, MCG
Grains				
Barley, cooked	0	0	3	36
Brown rice, cooked	0	0	1.1	14
Millet, cooked	0	0	1.3	2
Oatmeal, cooked	0	0	0.2	19
Wheat germ, 2 tbsp	0	0	2.6	11.4
Whole wheat bread, 1 slice	0	0	0.3	10
Legumes				
Black beans, cooked	0	10	1	2
Black-eyed peas, cooked	1	20	0.5	4
Garbanzo beans, cooked	2	28	2	6
Kidney beans, cooked	2	3	0.4	2
Lentils, cooked	3	11	1.2	6
Pinto beans, cooked	4	2	1.6	12
Soybeans, cooked	3	10	3.4	13
Split peas, cooked	1	11	1.6	1
Tofu, firm	1	0	0.1	44
White beans, cooked	0	0	2	2
Nuts, Seeds, Oils				
Almonds, ½ oz, 2 tbsp, 12 nuts	0	0	3.8	1
Brazil nuts, ½ oz, 2 tbsp, 3 nuts	0	0	1	420

SERVING SIZE: 1 CUP, RAW, UNLESS SPECIFIED	VITAMIN, C, MG*	BETA-CAROTENE MCG†	VITAMIN E, MG	SELENIUM, MCG
Grains *continued*				
Cashews, ½ oz, 2 tbsp	0	0	1	2
Flaxseed, 1 tbsp	1	0	0.1	6
Olive oil, 1 tsp	0	0	0.6	0
Peanuts, ½ oz, 2 tbsp, 17 nuts	0	0	1.1	1
Sunflower seeds, 1 tbsp	0	3	5	5
Walnuts, ½ oz, 2 tbsp, 7 halves	3	0	0.4	0.6
Other				
Cola	0	0	0	0
White sugar	0	0	0	1

*mg=milligram, 1/1,000 gram; *mcg=microgram, 1/1,000,000 gram

Getting the Protection You Need

Look at the table on pages 50–53 for the best sources of antioxidants. The daily recommended targets should be considered minimums. Somewhat higher intakes will do even more good in battling those free radicals. Vitamin-rich foods are preferable to supplements, which should be used with caution, because there is uncertainty about how these high intakes of antioxidants behave in the body. There are, in fact, upper limits to how much you should use from supplements. These have been set at 2,000 milligrams for vitamin C, 1,000 milligrams for vitamin E, and 200 micrograms for selenium. It is best to avoid beta-carotene supplements, as they do not appear to offer the same benefit as beta-carotene-rich foods.

More Cancer Fighters in Plant Foods

Selenium, beta-carotene, and vitamins E and C introduce you to the world of antioxidants, and the plant kingdom offers many more protective substances, from the bioflavonoids in the white part of citrus fruit to the catechins in green tea. Why do plants carry these protective chemicals? They serve as plants' natural shields from viruses, bacteria, and fungi. As we eat them, they will protect us, too, from many diseases, including cancers. Beyond beta-carotene and the other protectors we have already met, there is a delectable bunch of anticancer champions.

A leader among the fighting forces is garlic. Along with its botanical relatives—chives, leeks, onions, and scallions—it creates aromatic scents that fill the kitchen as you cook. These aromas actually come from sulfur compounds that work to disable toxic substances in your body. They block carcinogens from reaching their targets, destroy cancer cells, and suppress tumor growth. Garlic and onions have proven effectiveness against stomach and colorectal cancers, decreasing risk by as much as 50 to 60 percent when eaten regularly. Both are packed with protective compounds, and they work whether raw or cooked. One way to get maximum benefit from garlic is to chop it, leave it for ten to fifteen minutes, then add it to soups, stews, and savory dishes near the end of the cooking time. Contact with air improves the effectiveness of its cancer-fighting compounds. For tasty ways to add garlic and onions to your menus, try red pepper hummus, minestrone, or black bean chili. (See the recipe section for many delicious ideas.)

Certain herbs and spices can be cancer fighters, too. Special compounds called terpinoids give both flavor and cancer prevention qualities to caraway, cardamom, coriander, and celery seed as well as dill, lemongrass, mint, and spearmint. Rosemary and sage both contain antioxidants and have shown antitumor activity. Ginger contains a group of antioxidants that are even more potent than vitamin E. Turmeric, the spice that gives a yellow color to curries, is a relative of ginger and has been shown to block the growth of tumor calls. And there's good news for licorice lovers. Licorice may have some of the same benefits as soy and flax, protecting against breast cancer.

A Colorful Crew of Allies

Broccoli deserves special mention. It is rich in antioxidants and a good source of calcium, folate, and fiber (whose anticancer actions are covered later in this chapter). Broccoli is part of the botanical family known as cruciferous vegetables. With a meal of broccoli or cauliflower, we dine on the flowers of plants in this family. With cabbage or Brussels sprouts we eat the buds, and with kale, the leaves. All these veggies contain special compounds that block carcinogens from working their mischief. They are particularly effective against colorectal and thyroid cancers, but act against many other forms of cancer as well.

The red hue of tomatoes, watermelon, and strawberries is lycopene (another carotenoid). In a large Harvard study of health professionals, men who ate tomatoes or tomato products every day decreased their prostate cancer risk by 35 percent, compared to those who ate less than 1.5 servings a week. We absorb lycopene even better from tomatoes that have been heated, making spaghetti sauce, canned tomatoes, and tomato paste excellent sources. Perhaps all that sugary ketchup has some redeeming value after all! (But put it on a veggieburger instead of greasy fries.)

Green, leafy vegetables don't only boost your calcium intake; they also can go a long way toward cutting your risk of cancer. Greens contain the B vitamin folic acid, whose name comes from the word "foliage." Folic acid repairs breaks that can occur in the genetic material. In study after study, whether in the United States, Norway, Italy, China, or elsewhere, greens have shown their effectiveness against cancers of the colon, lungs, breast, and other sites.

Do you love blueberries on your cereal? Enjoy blueberry cornmeal muffins? Like a blueberry soy milk smoothie? These tasty berries may be one of the world's most protective foods. They neutralize free radicals that could otherwise damage your DNA. The U.S. Department of Agriculture's Center for Aging at Tufts University studied more than forty fruits and vegetables, measuring the effectiveness of each as an antioxidant. Blueberries ranked highest of all. Not only do they contain plenty of antioxidants, they also have the added cancer-fighting clout of anthocyanins, which give the blue color.

Here are some colorful foods rich in special protective substances along with fiber, antioxidants, vitamins, and minerals.

A RAINBOW OF HEALTH IN YOUR SHOPPING CART OR GARDEN

COLORS	FOODS	COLORFUL PROTECTIVE SUBSTANCES AND POSSIBLE ACTIONS
Red	Tomatoes and tomato products	Lycopene: antioxidant, cuts prostate cancer risk
Orange	Carrots, yams, sweet potatoes, mangoes	Beta-carotene: supports immune system and powerful antioxidant
Yellow-orange	Citrus fruits—oranges, lemons, grapefruit, papaya, peaches	Vitamin C, flavonoids: inhibit tumor cell growth, detoxify harmful substances
Green	Spinach, kale, collards, and other greens	Folate: builds healthy cells and genetic material
Green or white cruciferous vegetables	Broccoli, Brussels sprouts, cabbage, cauliflower	Indoles, lutein: eliminates excess estrogen and carcinogens
Green or white onion family	Garlic, onions, chives, and asparagus	Allyl sulfides: destroy cancer cells, reduce cell division, support immune system
Blue	Blueberries, purple grapes, plums	Anthocyanins: destroy free radicals
Red-purple	Grapes, berries, plums	Reservatrol: may decrease estrogen production
Brown	Whole grains, legumes	Fiber: carcinogen removal

With these foods you'll do more than protect yourself from cancer. In a study of eleven thousand health-conscious people, it was found that eating fruit daily cut deaths by 25 percent and stroke deaths by a full third. Unlike drug treatments, there are no unpleasant side effects.

Legumes: Protein Powerhouses of the Plant Kingdom

Earlier in this chapter, we looked at two major food groups—vegetables and fruits—with cancer-fighting properties. Legumes, including beans, peas, and lentils of every variety, as well as soy products, are the third major food group. Botanically, legumes are seeds that grow in pods. They are excellent sources of protein, without the saturated fat and cholesterol of animal products. They are also among our richest sources of fiber, and provide numerous other protective substances including folic acid, phytate, and phytoestrogens. There are more than fourteen thousand varieties. Here are a few favorites, in dishes from around the world:

- European lentil-barley stew
- Asian tofu dishes
- Mexican spicy pinto beans
- Indian chickpea curry
- Middle Eastern chickpea hummus
- Italian minestrone with kidney or white beans
- Central and South American black bean chili
- North African fava beans
- American-style soyburgers and dogs

For restaurant meals, here are good choices:

- bean, spinach, or vegetable burritos in Mexican restaurants
- tofu and mung bean sprouts in dishes at Asian restaurants
- falafel or hummus in Lebanese cafés
- dal or other spiced bean dishes in East Indian restaurants
- bean salads, bean or pea soups at Italian restaurants or at salad bars
- veggieburgers

The Joy of Soy Foods

Hormone-related cancers are far less common in Japan and China than in Western countries. Breast cancer is only a fourth as likely to occur in a Japanese woman, compared with an American woman. For men, prostate cancer rates are also much higher in the United States than in Japan. Part of the credit is given to the use of soy in place of animal products. Similarly, in Singapore, women of child-bearing age who used plenty of soy were found to have only 40 percent the risk of breast cancer, compared with women in the same region who did not.

Soy contains a number of compounds with anticancer action. Perhaps the best studied are phytoestrogens, very weak plant versions of the hormone estrogen. Though they are similar in structure, phytoestrogens have only about one one-thousandth the potency of human estrogen. They can displace human hormones at certain spots in the body, blocking their action and reducing cancer risk.

Here's how phytoestrogens seem to work: Excess human hormones are a driving force behind certain cancers. When estrogen attaches itself to breast tissue, it can increase cell division, driving the cancer process. However, when soy phytoestrogens bind to these sites, they displace some of your own estrogens, reducing their tendency to stimulate cancer growth. Picture each cell with a certain number of "seats" designed specifically to accommodate estrogen. Plant compounds that resemble estrogen fit quite nicely into these seats. Human estrogen is left with fewer seats to occupy. The result: Estrogen cannot exert its cancer-promoting effects.

Phytoestrogens have been shown to depress growth of cancer cells and help damaged cells either return to normal or self-destruct. They may stop the growth of blood vessels that tumors need to grow; halt the growth of breast, prostate, colon, and skin cancer cells; and block metastasis of breast and prostate cancer. As antioxidants, they protect DNA and cell membranes. Soybeans, tofu, soy milk, and other soy products contain appreciable amounts of phytoestrogens.

It may be that the subtle hormone effects of phytoestrogens from tofu, soy milk, and other soyfoods eaten in childhood bring benefits to women later in life. Research shows that they delay puberty slightly and lengthen the menstrual cycle after girls enter puberty.

For a woman in Japan, the average length of a menstrual cycle is four to six days longer than that of a Western woman, and the Japanese woman will have fewer cycles in her lifetime. This reduces the number of midcycle surges of estrogen into her body. The result is less overall exposure to estrogen and less risk of breast cancer.

In one study, Western women were fed 1½ to 2 servings of soyfoods each day, containing 45 milligrams of soy phytoestrogens. As a result, they developed longer menstrual cycles. Over a lifetime, this could be expected to decrease exposure to estrogen.

Men benefit from soy, too. Soy users in Asia and the United States have been shown to have lower cancer rates. Substances in soy have been shown to discourage growth of prostate cancer cells. In one study, high intakes of soy milk for a month led to a drop in hormone-related compounds that may be related to cancer growth.

Soy could well be the most versatile food in existence, taking on such different disguises that you wouldn't recognize that they all came from the same bean. At breakfast, scrambled tofu is great in a high-protein, cholesterol-free alternative to scrambled eggs. Delicious brands of soy milk are good in tea, on cereal, and in baking. (Choose fortified varieties.) For lunch try a veggieburger or a hot dog. At dinnertime try a tamale pie made with a soy-based veggie "meat," a spinach and mushroom fritatta (with tofu), or edamame (whole soybeans). Vegetarian and Asian restaurants have many soy options. Finish your meal with soy ice cream, pumpkin pie, or blueberry pudding. (See the recipe section.) As you can see, it's easy to fit servings of soyfoods into your day.

One situation where soy may be less desirable is for postmenopausal women who have already been diagnosed with breast cancer. Soy's abilities to exert even minor estrogenlike effects may be a disadvantage here, though the research hasn't given a clear message yet.

Nuts and Seeds: A Little Go a Long Way

Do you think of nuts and seeds as purely fattening snack foods? Three quarters of the calories in nuts and seeds come from fat. However, there are important differences between the fats in whole plant foods, and those in other high-fat foods such as meat and milk, processed foods made with hydrogenated oils, and refined vegetable oils. Nuts and seeds are loaded with antioxidants and other protective substances. They provide valuable plant protein and fiber. The bulk of their fat is a healthy combination of monounsaturated and polyunsaturated fats (including essential fatty acids), which help us absorb and use their protective substances.

The fat in animal products is another story. Meat and milk are high in saturated fat and cholesterol, whereas nuts and seeds are low in saturated fat and are cholesterol-free. The fat composition of nuts and seeds also bears little resemblance to the hydrogenated fats used in snack foods and many other products. These fats are laden with damaging trans fatty acids, which are made by a chemical process in which liquid oils are turned solid, producing molecules in unnatural shapes. Finally, when compared to refined oils, which have been stripped of beneficial components, nuts and seeds provide an abundance of protective substances, just as nature intended.

While it is important to limit total fat in the diet, the small amount of fat we do consume should come from whole plant foods. Generally about 10 to 15 percent of the calories in plant foods come from natural oils. Since nuts and seeds are much higher in fat, the key is to keep your portion sizes of these foods small. Add a spoonful of ground flaxseed to your morning cereal, spread a little almond butter on your toast instead of margarine, or sprinkle a few walnuts on your salad.

Cashews are particularly rich in zinc, almonds in calcium, flax and many other seeds in magnesium. A single Brazil nut contains more than double your recommended selenium intake for the day.

Flaxseeds for Omega-3s

Flaxseed oil and ground flaxseeds are particularly good choices because they are so high in essential omega-3 fatty acids. Omega-3 fatty acids help build cell membrane and support the immune system. They may also compete with "bad" fats that promote cancer.

You'll easily get your day's supply of omega-3 fatty acids from 1 teaspoonful of flaxseed oil or a tablespoonful of ground flaxseed. To protect it from oxygen damage, flaxseed oil must be stored in the refrigerator or the freezer. Use a little in dressings for salads or baked potatoes. Don't try to cook with this oil, however, as heat damages its omega-3s.

Ground seeds are a very good choice because in addition to omega-3s, they provide potent anticarcinogens called lignans, which may be particularly effective against the hormone-related cancers, acting in ways similar to soy. For you to absorb what you need from the seeds, they must be ground. Whole flaxseeds would carry on right through your digestive system, and out. To use flaxseed, grind it fresh in a spice or coffee grinder. You may also grind a cup every week or so and store it in the freezer. A spoonful can be added to a smoothie or sprinkled on breakfast cereal, a salad, or other dish. Ground flaxseed makes an excellent egg replacer in pancakes and muffin recipes. To make a "flax egg" for use in any recipes of this type, just mix 1 tablespoonful of ground flaxseed with 3 tablespoonfuls of water. Within a minute you'll see it thicken to an egglike consistency.

Great Grains and Friendly Fiber

Grains are the seeds of grasses. They have been a mainstay of human diets for ten thousand years. To the cultural melting pot of North America, rice and millet were introduced from Asia, oats and rye from Europe, barley from the Mediterranean and the Orient, while corn, quinoa, and amaranth are native to the Americas. Buck-wheat, actually a member of the rhubarb family, is a commonly used grain in Russia. Trying out new grains can be your ticket to a culinary tour of the world.

Grains provide more than half of the world's protein. They are packed with minerals, lots of B vitamins, protective compounds, and fiber. You'll want to choose whole grains because the milling process that turns whole grains into white flour or white rice removes the bran and the germ. From a commercial standpoint, refining increases shelf life, but the nutritional losses are immense. When wheat is refined, 95 percent of the protective phytonutrients are lost. In enriched white flour, iron and a few B vitamins have been added back, but the antioxidants selenium and vitamin E are not. Nor are magnesium, zinc, chromium, boron, potassium, manganese, several B vitamins, essential fats, and fiber.

Carbohydrates—Friend or Foe?

Have you heard nasty rumors about carbohydrates—that they make you fat, or put your blood sugar on a roller-coaster ride? These accusations should be aimed squarely at refined starchy foods and sugar. Such foods are absorbed quickly and give you a surge of calories, but they don't have staying power. They are a bit like stuffing the fire with paper. There's a big flare-up, and then it quickly drops down. The calories they provide also can be stored as fat when eaten in large quantities.

The story is quite different for whole grains. The energy in whole grains is an excellent fuel and is accompanied by many nutrients that our bodies need. These high-fiber foods are like slow-burning logs. Your body makes use of this energy very gradually throughout the day, keeping you on track for weight maintenance.

Although refined foods can lead to high blood sugar levels and high levels of the hormone insulin, which may speed up cell division and increase risk of cancer, whole grains are different. They provide energy without the peaks and valleys in energy and blood glucose. This is one way that fiber may protect against colon and breast cancer. An Italian study showed that use of refined grains increased colon cancer risk by 50 percent and rectal cancer by 30 percent. So when you think about carbohydrates, it makes a big difference whether you're talking about doughnuts, white bread, and croissants—or a healthy bowl of lentil barley soup.

Fiber: An Effective Force

There is no doubt about it. Fiber is on your side when it comes to fighting cancer. It fills you up and cleans you out. To top it off, it captures and eliminates nasty dietary components that can promote cancer. As far as allies go, this one's a keeper.

The fiber molecule itself is actually made up of an assortment of long chains of sugar and sugarlike molecules. The bonds that join these molecules resist digestion by enzymes in our intestines, allowing fiber to pass right through the stomach and the upper part of the intestine without being absorbed. Fiber-rich foods give a feeling of fullness by adding bulk and taking the place of foods that are very fattening, helping you to maintain a healthy body weight. It is found only in plants, never in foods from animal sources.

Fiber Removes Toxins

As we saw earlier, fiber does us a great service by carrying toxic substances out of the body. In addition to removing excess hormones and cholesterol, fiber helps carry away digestive juices that could otherwise be changed into toxic substances that encourage cells that line the colon to multiply out of control.

Across North America, colon cancer is the second most common cancer for women after breast cancer, and the third most common cancer for men after lung and prostate cancers. Yet a dietary shift toward more plant foods can make a big difference. As fiber intake rises, the risk of colorectal cancer drops, according to a study of more than twelve thousand men in seven countries over a twenty-five-year period. With an increase of 10 grams of fiber daily, the death rate from colorectal cancer decreased by 33 percent.

Healthy Digestion

The intestines are populated by millions of bacteria of different types. Some bacteria that enter our systems can make us sick. Others are "friendly" bacteria, good working partners to keep us in good health. Naturally, our food choices can make quite a difference in which bacteria thrive and which move out. Friendly bacteria need the fiber that manages to reach the lower intestine. They are particularly fond of types of fiber called resistant starch and oligosaccharides that come to us in whole grains, vegetables, and beans. In turn, these bacteria produce short-chain fatty acids that support the health of cells along the lining of the colon, preventing them from turning into out-of-control, quickly multiplying cancer cells.

A typical fiber intake in North America is dangerously low—between 11 and 13 grams a day. In the seven-countries study described above, researchers advised that for an effective defense against colorectal cancer, we may need average intakes of 40 or more grams of fiber a day.

Here's a typical American menu that is far too low in fiber:

Breakfast: two slices of bacon and an egg with one piece of buttered white toast, orange juice, and coffee with milk

Lunch: hamburger with tomato, lettuce, and mustard, small fries, and a milk shake

Dinner: a 3-ounce chicken breast, corn, white rice, and an iceberg lettuce side salad with Italian dressing

Adding it up, the total fiber is only 10 grams, not nearly enough for cancer protection.

Here are some better choices:

Breakfast: Oatmeal with raisins and soy milk, half a whole-wheat bagel with cashew or peanut butter, orange juice, and tea

Lunch: Veggieburger with lettuce, tomato, and mustard, with minestrone soup

Dinner: Thai Vegetables (see recipe page 188) over brown rice, with a berry cobbler

With these choices, fiber intake comes to a much healthier 32 grams.

Making these small (and delicious) changes easily triples your daily fiber intake. Choosing fiber-rich snack foods, such as a fruit smoothie made of strawberries, soy milk, and a banana, will boost your fiber by another 8 grams or so. Smoothies also are a great way to add cancer-fighting flax to your diet. Just sprinkle a spoonful of ground seeds in the blender with any of your favorite berries, juices, or nondairy milks. Remember to keep the flaxseeds refrigerated after use.

Fiber may have been made popular by the cereal manufacturers, but natural fiber is actually found in all varieties of vegetables, fruits, and beans.

Fiber Fights Colon Cancer

Colon cancer starts when cells along its inner lining start to change. Initially, small growths, called polyps, form on the colon lining. These polyps are not cancerous and do not spread to other parts of the body. However, they are a sign that something is amiss. Eventually, overgrowing cells become cancerous, invading the colon wall and spreading to other parts of the body.

Fiber changes this course of events. Fiber hampers the action of cancer-causing agents and escorts them out of the body. Fiber also supports a healthy environment for the cells along the intestine, so that cell division doesn't get out of control.

Fiber also fights breast cancer. As we have seen, too much estrogen over the years, from fatty diets and hormone replacement therapy, can be a driving force in promoting cancer. Luckily, your body can use fiber to rid itself of excess estrogen. As we saw in chapter 3, excess estrogen is excreted in bile that passes from the liver into the intestine. When fiber is abundant in the diet, it sweeps the intestines clean instead of allowing the estrogen to be reabsorbed. Together, fiber and estrogen pass on out of the body with the wastes. Vegetarian women, whose diets are high in fiber, have much less of this potentially damaging estrogen circulating in their blood.

Fiber is a winner in weight management as well. Severely overweight women have much greater risk of breast cancer compared with lean women, and the likelihood increases with age. Being overweight and having too many years of exposure to estrogen are both very important factors in the development of endometrial cancer, too. Again, fiber-rich plant foods, with their many benefits, can be a lifesaver.

All plant foods contain substances that protect us from disease. As research unfolds, we discover that more and more of them have potent anticancer activity in the form of fiber, antioxidants, and a host of other compounds yet to be fully understood. With a varied, plant-based diet, we create a powerful defense against cancer and support ourselves in vibrant health.

5

Foods for
Cancer Survival

So far we have seen that foods are vital for preventing cancer. But a growing body of scientific research also shows that foods can play a decisive role *even after cancer has been diagnosed.* Certainly, surgery, radiation, chemotherapy, and other treatments are important. But the foods we put on our plates for breakfast, lunch, and dinner may well be our most essential allies.

Nutrition works in several ways. First, your body's principal anticancer defense is your immune system, made up of specialized white blood cells that patrol your bloodstream to seek out and destroy cancer cells. Their strength depends on the foods you eat. Second, foods influence hormones. If your diet is planned the right way, you can target the hormones that promote cancer growth and cut them down to size. Third, if you are undergoing cancer treatment, the right foods can support you on the road to getting well.

Many of the findings in this area are new. But the fact is, scientists have long suspected that foods play a major role in cancer survival. In the early 1960s, Dr. Ernst Wynder, who had been one of the medical pioneers who uncovered the role of tobacco in lung cancer, among other discoveries, was struck by a surprising finding in Japan. Not only were Japanese women much more likely than American or European women to stay free of breast cancer, but also, when it did strike, they were much more likely to survive.

In teasing apart the various reasons why this might be so, the explanation that emerged most strongly related to the traditional Japanese diet. Low in fat and high in vegetables, grains, and the natural cancer-fighting compounds they hold, this diet worked almost like a medicine. By analyzing the diets that seem to hold power against cancer, Dr. Wynder and other researchers set out to find new tools to fight the disease.

Their search paid off. In this chapter we will look at the scientific studies that have shown how foods can strengthen your defenses. But before we start, a few cautions: First, now is not the time to simply dabble with a few diet changes. While healthy people might only be willing to make minor adjustments to their diet to avert illness in the seemingly distant future, if you have cancer already, you will want to take things more seriously. When we are diagnosed with cancer, we can no longer pretend that we have some sort of magical protection—genetic or otherwise—against the disease. Now is the time to pull out all the stops. You'll want to put to work everything we know about choosing protective foods.

Second, work with your doctor. For many people, surgery or other treatments are essential, and the anticancer approaches available to us are broader every day. Use diet with other treatments, not in place of them.

Third, do not get stuck in denial. So many people say, "I had cancer, but I was operated on and my surgeon got the whole thing. I'm cured!" With those reassuring words, we imagine we can happily return to the very habits that may have encouraged cancer in the first place. The fact is, your doctor has no idea if he or she "got the whole thing." A tumor can quietly seed cancer cells into your bloodstream long before you are ever wheeled into the operating room. These cells can lurk in other organs for years before beginning to grow once again. So you will want to use foods to give your body every chance to eliminate these unwanted cells.

Setting Blame Aside

People with cancer sometimes feel that if foods may play a role in causing cancer or fostering its growth, then they are somehow to blame for their disease. It is as if every new research study on nutrition points a finger of culpability. If you have found yourself feeling this way, let me encourage you to set blame aside. First of all, no one could have known in advance what these studies would show. We and our families ate the foods we believed to be healthy, as far as we knew at the time. If we have better information now, that is all to the good. Second, it is easy to get cancer. Even if you've taken good care of yourself, your cancer risk does not drop to zero, just as some people who take tremendous risks, such as chronic smoking, never get the disease.

Jack Nicklaus used to say that you can spend all day trying to figure out how your golf ball got into the woods—or you can just go in and get it out. Whatever combination of genetic, environmental, and dietary factors came together to cause cancer, now is the time to fight back.

Foods and Immune Defenses

Some people use visual imagery to bolster their cancer treatments. They imagine white blood cells traveling through the bloodstream, finding the cancer, and methodically attacking it. Each voracious white blood cell gobbles up one cancer cell after another, eliminating these intruders and returning the body to health.

You can do more than simply imagine this process. You can power it up. By avoiding some foods and adding others, you will give your immune cells new strength. The fact is, one of the reasons why cancer occurs more often as people get older may simply be that our immune strength has started to flag. As we reach middle age and beyond, our immune cells are not the stalwart soldiers they once were. But you can change that. By giving your white blood cells better rations, so to speak, you can return these out-of-shape defenders to fighting form.

Cutting Fat and Cholesterol

First, your white blood cells cannot work in an oil slick. It is essential to get the fat out of your diet. Researchers have conducted many different studies, feeding various high-fat and low-fat diets to volunteers, and have even gone so far as to drip fat into their veins with intravenous lines. Over and over, they have found that reducing the fat content of the diet gives white blood cells more power, while high-fat diets weaken them.

Researchers in New York asked a group of volunteers to cut the fat from their diets—both animal fats and vegetable oils—for three months. They had been getting about 40 percent of their calories from fat, which is fairly typical of Americans, and now it was to be cut to 20 percent. The researchers then took blood samples and examined the white blood cells' ability to recognize and destroy cancer cells. The diet change clearly worked. Reducing fat in the diet rejuvenated the white blood cells. And those who cut their fat intake the most had the strongest cancer-fighting cells. As you know by now, the healthiest diets eliminate animal fats completely and keep vegetable oils modest.

Also as you know by now, you do need a small amount of fat in your diet. But the amount you need is minuscule, much less than most people get. There is no need at all for animal fats in the diet, and you are better off without them. By also avoiding fried foods and added vegetable oils, you can easily reduce your fat content dramatically.

A 200-Year-Old "Breakthrough"

"Dr. John Bell, who was, about a hundred years ago, professor in a leading college in London, wrote that a careful adherence to a vegetarian dietary tended to prevent cancer. He also stated that in some cases persons who had already acquired cancer had been cured by the adherence to a non-flesh dietary. When I first read this book, I did not agree with the author; I thought he was mistaken; but I have gradually come to believe that what he says on this subject is true."

DR. JOHN HARVEY KELLOGG, 1903

Cholesterol has long been vilified by doctors for its role in heart problems, and for good reason. The more cholesterol there is coursing through your veins, the more likely you are to have a heart attack. However, cholesterol also affects your immunity. In test-tube studies, researchers have found that, in excess, cholesterol weakens the cell membranes that are your white blood cells' suits of armor.

Lowering your cholesterol level is easier than you might have imagined. By shifting your diet from animal products to foods from plant sources and cutting the fat—which you wanted to do anyway—you are likely to reduce your cholesterol level significantly.

Natural Immune Boosters

Certain foods can boost your immune system's ability to destroy cancer cells, even at various stages after their development. Researchers have added various foods or supplements to volunteers' diets and then checked their immune strength, while other research teams have added specific nutrients to white blood cells in the test tube. The results showed that the four antioxidant superstars we learned about earlier are still our best defense.

As we saw earlier, studies have shown that a diet providing sufficient levels of beta-carotene—easy to get in a couple of carrots or a even sweet potato pancakes—per day clearly boosts immune strength. However, beta-carotene supplements are not the same as beta-carotene-rich foods. In a disturbing research on smokers, beta-carotene pills did not help them at all. Smokers, of course, are at very high risk of lung cancer, and those whose diets are high in beta-carotene-rich foods do, in fact, have a measure of protection. But when smokers take beta-carotene pills, their cancer rates are actually *higher* than without them. In other words, where vitamin-rich foods help, vitamin pills may not.

The moral of the story is that nature packs vitamins into foods in intricate combinations that pills cannot replicate. A beta-carotene supplement gives you nothing but beta-carotene. On the other hand, vegetables and fruits contain hundreds of different carotenoids, which have biological power of their own. You will find it not only in carrots and sweet potatoes but also in other yellow-orange foods such as butternut squash and even in green vegetables such as spinach, broccoli, and kale, although its orange color is hidden by the deep green of their chlorophyll.

A study of elderly men and women showed that the more vitamin E they had in their blood, the stronger their immunity. Vitamin E protects cells from free radicals and helps maintain a healthy immune system. But once again, it is better to choose the right foods instead of supplements. High doses can actually suppress immunity. In a study of teenagers and young adults, researchers found that taking just 300 milligrams of vitamin E daily—which is less than you'll find in some supplements—impaired their white blood cells' ability to knock out bacteria. Other studies have shown much the same thing: A little is good, a lot is not necessarily better.

Healthy vitamin E sources include sweet potatoes, brown rice, and beans such as chickpeas, navy beans, and soy products. Nuts are rich in vitamin E and also a little rich in fat, so you'll want to eat them only occasionally.

Vitamin C is known for its ability to fight free radicals and bolster immune strength, so you'll want to include it every day, whether you're in tip-top shape or battling an illness. In the bargain, it also keeps your vitamin E working well—that is, as vitamin E molecules are used up in the course of fighting free radicals, vitamin C repairs them and returns them to action. There is plenty of vitamin C in fruits, of course, but you'll also find surprisingly large amounts in broccoli, Brussels sprouts, and many other vegetables.

You'll recall that selenium is a mineral naturally found in the soil. Plants draw it in through their roots and pack it into their cells, where it acts to protect them from free radicals. If you eat these plants, their selenium will protect you, too. However, selenium also is an immune-booster. You'll find it in the whole grains that are used to make breads, cereals, and some pastas.

Okay, so if we cut the fat and cholesterol, and boost our intake of vegetables, fruits, and whole grains to take advantage of their natural immune boosters, will we see an effect? No question. Researchers at the German Cancer Research Center in Heidelberg decided to look at people following healthy vegetarian diets, and compared them to nonvegetarian volunteers working at the cancer center. They drew blood samples and tested their white blood cells' ability to knock out cancer cells. The results were striking: The vegetarians had more than double the ability to destroy cancer cells, compared to nonvegetarians. You can do better still, because, while many of these vegetarians had not yet eliminated dairy products or eggs and some were having only fairly modest vegetable portions, you can take these added steps for even more immune power. Cancer drugs are truly miraculous, but so are the medicines that grow from the ground and hang from the trees. For anyone facing cancer at any stage, it would be prudent to take full advantage of nature's full range of immunity-boosting foods.

The Example of Breast Cancer

To apply these findings to your life and that of your loved ones, let's start with a look at how nutrition affects breast cancer survival, both because it occurs so frequently and also because it illustrates principles that apply to other forms of the disease.

In many studies, researchers have tracked how diet adjustments can help people with breast cancer. The benefits first show up in blood tests. For example, cutting down on fat reduces the amount of estrogen in the blood, which is critical, since estrogens fuel breast cancer growth, as we saw in chapter 4. The effect is quick. Researchers at the National Cancer Institute found that when women cut their fat intake from near 40 percent to 20 percent of calories, the amount of estrogen in their blood quickly dropped by 17 percent. Dropping fat even farther leads to much greater changes. The result is that there is less estrogen to promote the growth and spread of cancer.

Cutting the fat and increasing fiber also increase sex-hormone-binding globulin (SHBG), the protein that harnesses estrogens in the bloodstream, reducing their ability to promote cancer cell growth. A low-fat, vegan diet increased the amount of SHBG in the blood by 19 percent in just five weeks. In turn, SHBG tames estrogen's effects.

It helps, not only to avoid fatty animal products such as meats and whole milk, but also to steer clear of even low-fat animal products such as skim milk. Not only are these foods devoid of protective fiber and vitamin C, but also researchers have found that skim milk has the untoward effect of boosting the amount of insulin-like growth factor I (IGF-I) in the bloodstream, apparently because of its load of protein and sugars. IGF-I is a stimulus for cancer cell growth, and milk drinkers have approximately 10 percent more IGF-I circulating in their blood compared to people who consume little or no milk.

The benefits of healthier diets are clear, not only in these laboratory tests but also in studies of actual people with cancer. In Buffalo, New York, researchers examined the diets of women who had been diagnosed with breast cancer and followed them over the next several years to see how they did. They found that a woman's risk of dying at any point in time increased 40 percent for every 1,000 grams of fat she consumed per month. In practical terms this amount of fat is roughly the difference between a typical American diet, which piles up about 2,000 grams of fat a month, and a plant-based diet prepared with little or no added fat, which has fewer than 1,000 grams of fat per month. This does not mean that a person's risk of dying is 40 percent. It simply means that, in the higher-fat group, the risk is 40 percent higher than it would otherwise have been.

Similarly, a 1995 study of 698 postmenopausal breast cancer patients, followed for six years, showed that those who ate the least fat had only half the risk of dying, compared to the other women. A Canadian research study nailed down the specific type of fats of most concern, finding that a higher intake of saturated fats—the type found particularly in animal products—was linked to more aggressive cancers.

Cutting the fat from your diet gets your hormones into better balance. And it has another benefit, too: It helps you lose weight. Research shows that thinner women are not only less likely to develop cancer; if it occurs, they also are less likely to succumb to it. A change in the type of food you eat helps you lose weight in a healthy way without cutting calories or restricting portion sizes.

Countries with low cancer rates base their diets on staple grains such as rice or wheat noodles. The same diet pattern helps people survive cancer as well. A study of women who had been previously treated for breast cancer showed that a diet rich in grains (e.g., breads and cereals) cut recurrence risk in half. So include whole wheat toast or grainy muffins in your breakfast, or try tomorrow's lunch on whole wheat pita bread. You'll boost your health and feel full longer.

Tea vs. Cancer?

Green tea has long been said to have health benefits. In a study of 472 Japanese women with breast cancer, researchers found that women who drank more than 5 cups of green tea per day had a significant drop in their risk of a recurrence. The benefit was apparent for women who had had milder forms of the disease. How does it work? The credit seems to go to natural anticancer compounds in tea called polyphenols.

Cancers of the Uterus, Ovary, and Prostate

The uterus and the ovary are similar to the breast in that they are sensitive to estrogens. Just as high-fat, animal-product-based diets are linked to higher breast cancer rates, the same is true for uterine and ovarian cancer. Unfortunately, the role of diet in cancer survival has not been as well studied for these forms of the disease. Nonetheless, building your diet from vegetables, fruits, grains, and legumes, while avoiding fatty foods, will likely tend to reduce estrogen's cancer-promoting effect.

For prostate cancer, similar considerations apply, except that we are concerned about the hormone testosterone, instead of estrogen. There is good reason to believe that foods can not only influence the risk that prostate cancer will begin, but also whether it progresses. Cancer cells arise in the prostates of middle-aged and older men surprisingly often. If these cells simply stay put, they cause no problem. They are as dormant as seeds on dry soil. It is only when they begin to multiply and invade neighboring tissues or spread through the bloodstream that serious problems arise.

Many prostate cancer researchers are convinced that diet's most important role is not in stopping cancer from starting, but in determining whether it will stay small or begin to grow and spread. Happily, the same diet changes—cutting fat and boosting fiber—that reduce estrogen do the same for testosterone.

Dr. Dean Ornish, the medical pioneer at the Preventive Medicine Research Institute who proved that lifestyle changes, including a low-fat vegetarian diet, regular exercise, and stress reduction could reverse existing heart disease, is now applying a similar regimen to prostate cancer. While the research is still ongoing at the time of this writing, early results are promising.

Other research studies have shown that men with more IGF-I in their bloodstreams are at higher risk of developing prostate cancer compared to other men, as we saw in chapter 4. But IGF-I is a potent stimulus for cancer cell growth. As we saw above, regular milk drinking raises IGF-I levels, and avoiding milk is associated with safer levels.

Digestive Tract Cancers

Diet changes also are important in digestive tract cancers—those arising in the mouth, esophagus, stomach, colon, rectum, or liver. Researchers have focused on changing the course of the disease in people who have precancerous conditions, and have identified a protective role for certain nutrients. The benefits of beta-carotene were studied in a group of men and women in Arizona who had pre-cancerous changes in their mouths (which doctors refer to with the technical name leukoplakia, which simply means "white spots"). These people were at high risk for oral cancer. The research team asked each of them to take 60-milligram beta-carotene supplements, the equivalent of four carrots, per day.

For many, the spots in their mouths regressed or disappeared. After six months the protective effect was so strong that even those who then discontinued the beta-carotene supplements still showed lingering protection a year later. As we saw earlier, however, you are better off getting your beta-carotene, along with hundreds of its relatives, from vegetables and fruits rather than pills.

High-fiber foods have shown their power as well. In the late 1980s, Jerome J. DeCosse, a surgeon at Cornell Medical Center, gave bran to patients with colon polyps. Polyps are often signs that colon cancer is around the corner. Six months later, he found that the polyps became smaller and fewer in number. Similar studies followed, showing fiber's benefits.

The best prescription for cancer patients, of course, is not found simply in vitamin pills, bran supplements, or the occasional whole wheat muffin. Grains, beans, fruits, and vegetables are loaded with vitamins, minerals, natural fiber, and other vital nutrients. The more of them you build into your diet, the better off you'll be.

6

Nutrition during Cancer Treatment

If you or a loved one is undergoing chemotherapy or other cancer treatments, you may find that eating is complicated by odd tastes, loss of appetite, nausea, or other problems. You'll need a bit of patience, but these annoyances will pass. In the meantime, here are some tips to help you.

Lack of Appetite

- Being relaxed helps, so you'll want to make mealtime calm and unhurried. If your appetite is intermittent, go ahead and eat whenever you are hungry. Let yourself have several small meals during the day instead of trying to get through three large ones.
- Morning may be the time you have the most appetite. If so, make the most of this time. For example, have two small meals and a snack before noon.
- Drink liquids half an hour before or after meals so you don't get filled up with fluid when you're trying to eat.

Taste Changes

Your sense of taste may change if you are on medications or receiving radiation treatment to the head or neck. Perhaps you can hardly taste or smell food at all. Nonetheless, keep eating during this temporary stage. Foods will still be nourishing.

Your sense of taste may continue to change during treatment. Experiment with sour, sweet, salty, and bitter foods to find out what's best for you. Try different seasonings.

Coping with Taste Changes

- For those with an increased sense of strong or bitter tastes, the mild flavor of some soy products can be a welcome change.
- For those with a metallic taste in their mouth, use plastic dishware and silverware.
- Peanut butter, tofu, and beans are bland foods that may be appealing.

If taste blindness is a problem, using marinades and seasonings for tofu and tempeh can enhance the flavor.

Dry Mouth

If you have persistent mouth dryness due, for example, to the effect of radiation on the glands that produce saliva, you may wish to sip water frequently or use a mouth spray. Meals will be easier with sauces or salad dressings, and you'll likely be using your blender more than ever before to create soups and fruit smoothies. Some people find that sugarless gum, especially citrus-flavored, helps moisten their mouths.

Chewing or Swallowing Problems

Anticancer drugs, radiation, and infection may result in tender gums, or a sore mouth or throat.

Try these tips:

- Choose soft foods that are easy to chew and swallow: oatmeal, Cream of Wheat, scrambled tofu, soup, mashed potatoes, blueberry pudding, or smoothies. (See the recipe section for ideas.) Bananas, watermelons, other soft fruits, applesauce, and fruit nectars are nutritious and go down easily.

- Mash or puree any variety of vegetable just as you would mashed potatoes. If you don't already have a food processor or blender, you'll find it's an excellent investment.
- Make sure that veggies and beans are well cooked, so they are soft and tender.
- Adding a vegan gravy can make foods easier to swallow.

Here are tips from a woman who appreciated her experience at the Block Medical Center in Illinois.

"I was extremely apprehensive about taking chemo, but in retrospect, I am glad that I did it. I think a good whole foods diet makes a huge difference, not only in how you feel, but also in how you respond to the treatment. Also the supplements I took, I believe, kept me strong throughout. I was able to continue working during that time. Every treatment gets easier, in part because you know what to expect, and also because the body tolerates it better. Here are some things I found to be extremely helpful:

1. Walk as much as you can. It makes a difference in how you feel during treatment and also makes it easier to sleep. (The fatigue is one of the worst side effects.)

2. Miso soup and tamari broth soups are wonderful for nausea. They work better than Zofran. During the last three rounds I didn't use it because the soup worked better.

3. Sparkling water helps a lot, too, to settle the stomach.

4. I ate lots of leafy vegetables, usually three times a day. Kale, collard greens, cabbage, broccoli, etc. I believe that they counteracted some of the negative effects of chemotherapy, and also helped clear it from my system."

M. L., Illinois

- Vegetables, beans, and grains, in just about any combination, can make a good soup. In fact, people can live on soups for months on end and never run out of new tastes and combinations.
- To boost the calories, add cashews or tofu. Use soft, medium, or firm tofu, or any silken tofu. They blend right in, give a lovely creaminess, and are a gentle form of nourishment.
- Backpacking equipment stores sell containers with lids that screw on tightly and don't leak a drop, making it simple to transport foods without having soup or a fruit shake spill in your bag.
- Blended drinks and smoothies can help you swallow pills if you find that thinner liquids don't work. Pills and supplements may need to be crushed and dissolved, or try a liquid formula instead.
- Certain foods can be irritating, such as those that are very sour, salty, spicy, or coarse-textured. This may not be the time for citrus fruits, raw vegetables, or toast.
- If swallowing is hard, tilt your head forward, sideways, or back to find a position that works better. You may need to eat with extra awareness so you don't choke on food. If you are afraid of choking, ask your healthcare provider to arrange an assessment and advice about the best textures and techniques for your situation.
- People treated for esophageal cancer or some stomach cancers may need to sit up for half an hour or so after meals.

A Helpful Hint

"When I can't finish a meal, even when I'm out for dinner, I package it up and blend it later. That way, there's something good to eat when I get hungry again. Everything might end up looking like pea soup, but it sure doesn't all taste like pea soup. I've made wonderful combinations."

JENISE, VANCOUVER

Nausea and Vomiting

Nausea can be a side effect of surgery, chemotherapy, radiation, immunotherapy, and of cancer itself.

Try these tricks:

- Foods that may help are oatmeal, mashed potatoes, smoothies, sherbet, and soft fruits such as canned peaches. You may sip a clear liquid such as miso soup or juice. Sucking on ice chips can help, too.
- Try eating dry foods such as toast, crackers, pretzels, or other dry foods before getting up and about every two hours.
- Eat a little, and often. Fasting can cause a drop in blood sugar that makes nausea even worse.
- You may find that you're extrasensitive to certain smells and textures. If possible, avoid being near food while it is being prepared or around foods with aromas you find unpleasant.
- Avoid greasy, spicy, supersweet, or fried foods. Choose cold or room-temperature foods.

Diarrhea

Diarrhea can be a side effect of treatment, or result from emotional upset, food sensitivity, or infections. If diarrhea is severe or lasts for several days, be sure to let your care provider know, because you could easily become dehydrated.

The following can be irritants or lead to diarrhea in other ways: caffeine, alcohol, fat, spices, and lactose (in milk and dairy products).

Try having small amounts throughout the day. Drink plenty of liquids in beverages, soups, and smoothies. Have these warm or at room temperature, instead of very hot or very cold.

Constipation

Some drugs used in treatment can result in constipation, as can too little water or a lack of fiber. The best prescription for constipation is water; fiber-rich foods; and, if you're up to it, exercise. Whole grains, beans, fruits, and vegetables will add helpful fiber. Natural laxatives are prunes, prune juice, rhubarb, and papaya.

Weight Loss

Sometimes treatment can cause unwanted weight loss. If you find you're just not getting enough calories from vegetables, fruits, grains, and legumes, add some healthier sources of fat such as nuts, avocados, or olives. In these plant foods, fats come packaged with antioxidants and are better for you than animal fat, pastries, sweets, or refined vegetable oils.

You also may lose muscle. For this, there's a three-part solution. First, rely on tofu, tempeh, and other protein-rich foods. Second, be sure to get enough calories. Third, include moderate amounts of physical activity, to the extent that you can, during and after treatment. This will help you put on muscle, not fat.

Make sure you have healthy snacks available, whether you're at home or away from home. Keep almonds, crackers, and fresh or dried fruit in your bag, briefcase, or glove compartment. Buy soy milk and tomato juice in individual portions so you can pack them along with you. You'll find tips for restaurant eating, traveling, and social events in this book as well.

Nutrient-Dense Snacks

- Dry beans and peas, nuts, peanut butter, and seeds are examples of foods commonly eaten by nonvegetarians, but perhaps not very often or in small quantities. These can be maximized to supply a greater percentage of calorie and protein requirements.
- Shakes can be made with soy milk, tofu, and nondairy frozen desserts, and can be flavored with fruit, chocolate syrup, or extracts to make a tasty, calorie-rich treat.
- Many varieties of trail mixes are readily available and are great for high-energy snacking.

Quick and Easy High-Calorie Snacks

- bean tacos/burritos
- fruit shakes
- nondairy frozen desserts
- soy yogurt, custards, and puddings
- peanut butter on crackers or fruit
- bean and chunky vegetable soups
- dried fruit, nuts, and seeds
- bagels

Weight Gain

If you're overweight, weight reduction is an excellent long-term goal. However, big changes in weight during treatment are not recommended. Right now, getting the nutritional support you need is top priority.

However, some chemotherapy drugs can cause unavoidable weight gain. After treatment, this weight can be lost, with physical activity and healthy food choices. You'll especially want to keep your fat intake low.

Eating during Recovery

Right after surgery, chemotherapy, or radiation, your body needs to recover strength, rebuild, and correct any problems that may have developed. The combination of good food and exercise, to the extent you are able, is vitally important.

Anemia can result from treatments, blood loss, or from cancer itself. Legumes and whole grains are great sources of iron to help prevent low iron stores. Eating vitamin C-rich foods along with these foods will help you absorb iron more efficiently. Avoiding dairy products is important, since they can interfere with iron absorption. Iron deficiency anemia is no more common among vegetarians than among meat eaters, so don't think you have to resume eating meat, even temporarily, to keep your iron level healthy.

Here are combinations that give you iron, vitamin C, and protein:

- a fruit smoothie with tofu
- crackers, peanut butter, and a glass of orange juice
- hummus with veggie sticks
- a stir-fry with tofu and vegetables
- a taco with beans, tomatoes, and sprouts (with or without avocado)
- soups that contain vegetables and beans or lentils
- Broccoli Burritos (see page 166)

Programs Offering Nutritional Support

The following are a few treatment programs you'll find in North America. They may direct you to cooking classes, medical support, or written materials for people undergoing cancer treatment. You will want to speak with your doctor about finding a program that meets your individual needs.

Block Medical Center, Evanston, Illinois, where Dr. Keith Block's cancer treatment program uses diet, nutritional pharmacology, and stress reduction in an advanced system of healing, with treatments tailored to each individual.

847-492-3040   www.BlockMD.com

CaP-CURE, the Association for the Cure of Cancer of the Prostate, in Santa Monica, California, provides resource materials and direction to current prostate treatment research programs in different parts of the country.

800-757-CURE or 310-458-2873   www.capcure.org/

Center for Integrated Healing, Vancouver, British Columbia, Canada, where support is given for plant-based nutrition and an integrated approach to healthcare that combines both conventional and complementary treatments.

604-734-3496   www.healing.bc.ca

Kushi Institute, in Becket, Massachusetts, is the leading macrobiotic center in North America. Macrobiotic diets are based on whole grains, vegetables (including sea vegetables), beans and soyfoods, fruits, nuts, seeds, and teas. Guidance is available on a diet that may support the medical treatment of your own physician.

800-975-8744 or 413-623-2322

www.macrobiotics.org/home.html
kushiinstitute.org

You can find a dietitian in your area via the Internet. If you are in the United States, go to www.eatright.org/find2.html and click Consumer Search. Then you can find a specialist in both oncology and vegetarian nutrition.

Go to www.dietitians.ca/diet/ASP/findadietitian.asp in Canada. Under Specialty click Vegetarian/Vegan Nutrition, and under Health click Cancer.

PART III

Lifelong Health

7

Putting Food Power
to Work against
Today's Common Cancers

By now it will come as no surprise that food choices and other habits can dramatically influence our risk for cancer, as we have touched upon in previous chapters. Let's put this to work.

Let's look at the most common cancers to see what science has taught us. Some of the observations are brand new, while others have been known for decades. In 1982, the National Research Council reviewed the mountain of important links between diet and cancer. In 1997, the World Cancer Research Fund and the American Institute for Cancer Research summarized the even stronger evidence and made recommendations for putting it to use. And continuing research is making many details clearer still. Here's what we know.

Lung Cancer

Whether you're shopping at a convenience store, reading a magazine, or attending a sports event, it's hard to escape the tobacco industry's heavy hand in the advertising game. There are people who do an outstanding job of luring us into giving cigarettes a try. Unfortunately, teenagers are the ones who often take the bait, ending up as lifelong smokers. Among their parents, there are those who have "quit" dozens of times, only to relapse again and again. It's a hard habit to break, apparent in the increase in lung cancer incidence and deaths around the world.

The best advice we can take is never to start. With that said, there will always be people who will ignore this advice, and there still will be nonsmokers who develop lung cancer due to exposure to X rays, radon gas, asbestos, air pollution, or other factors, so it doesn't hurt to put other safeguards to work.

Clearly, smokers have a greater risk for lung cancer than nonsmokers no matter what they eat. Delicate lung tissue is simply ill equipped to fend off the daily (or even occasional) onslaught of concentrated carcinogens delivered through cigarette smoke. If you have been held hostage by the smoking habit, it's never too late to quit. In just eight hours after your last cigarette, blood oxygen levels return to normal; after one smoke-free year, risk of coronary heart disease will be half that of a smoker's. Perhaps you've tried to go it alone and would benefit from the advice and assistance of your physician. There are dozens of programs available to help you, from nicotine patches to Internet "support groups." Just begin looking, and you're bound to find your way to a smoke-free existence.

However, despite the dangers of smoking, foods still have a protective effect. If a smoker or a nonsmoker has a choice between eating grilled vegetables over rice or a hamburger and fries for lunch, the vegetarian meal will provide much-needed antioxidants and even appears to offer some protection against smoking-related lung cancer.

Supersize Your Fruits and Veggies

Picture a banquet of orange and green foods. It might contain sweet potatoes, carrots, cantaloupes, pumpkins, squash, spinach, broccoli, zucchini, kale, and collard greens, to name just a few. When you include these in your daily diet, you're building a strong defense against lung cancer. All vegetables and fruits do the job, but green and orange vegetables and fruits, which are high in carotenoids, have been shown to decrease lung cancer risk in both men and women, smokers and nonsmokers. In addition to beta-carotene, it is believed that the vitamin C and folate they contain may be the muscle behind their strength. Despite some ambiguity regarding which specific nutrient deserves the credit, there is consensus that vegetables and fruits cut lung cancer risk.

With Big Gulp sodas and supersized fries on the menu, many of us eat far more than our parents did. If you want to nourish your body, you'll want to indulge in these about as often as birthday cake. But when your appetite is big, why not supersize your vegetable serving? Don't reach for a jumbo hot dog, which will fill you with fat and other cancer-promoting ingredients. Grab a veggieburger and pile it up with fresh tomatoes, lettuce, onions, or even some sautéed spinach. Try chunky, *baked* potato wedges, a large slice of melon, or a big glass of vegetable juice. You certainly don't have to cut back on flavor, variety, or even portions when you choose the right foods.

Not only are fruits and vegetables important in preventing lung cancer, they also improve the prognosis if it strikes. In Hawaii, nearly seven hundred men and women with lung cancer were asked about their dietary habits in the year before their diagnosis, their history of tobacco use, and other lifestyle and environmental conditions. Survival clearly improved with the increased consumption of certain fruits and vegetables. If particular components of vegetables and fruits can prolong survival in patients with lung cancer, you can imagine how industriously these little nutrients work on you (and in you) every day. All you've got to do is eat up! It's the most cost-effective and enjoyable step you can take.

Synthetic Shortcomings

It is important to understand that positive nutrient effects have been shown mainly with the consumption of vitamin- and mineral-rich *plant foods,* rather than with vitamin and mineral supplements. In fact, results from large, controlled trials of beta-carotene supplementation do not show benefits in lung cancer prevention. Instead, it had the opposite effect. Smokers with lung cancer succumbed more quickly to the disease after taking high doses of beta-carotene. The reason for this is not entirely clear. However, it may have to do with the fact that vegetables and fruits contain hundreds of different carotenoids, while beta-carotene pills give you only beta-carotene. The result may be an altered absorption of other carotenoids or perhaps other vitamins. So go natural, and let a nice variety of plant foods supply the perfect balance of nutrients.

Cut the Fat

New research studies have shown a clear pattern: Higher lung cancer rates are associated with greater fat intake. It appears that fat from the foods you eat acts as a sort of fertilizer on cancerous tumors, encouraging their growth and ability to spread, as well as impairing your immune defenses against them. In fact, the particles in the bloodstream that carry fat and cholesterol also escort chemical carcinogens from place to place in the body. We have long known that it's a good idea to minimize fat intake, and avoiding lung cancer is yet another reason.

One study, initiated in 1960 and conducted in seven countries, showed that high fat intake, particularly the saturated fat we find in animal products, was linked to lung cancer deaths. Cutting the fat is a necessary step, like clearing clogged pipes so fresh water can move through easily. By piling your plate with cancer-fighting veggies, your protection increases exponentially. Try making veggie lasagna with spinach, mushrooms, eggplant, and soy cheese instead of ground beef and mozzarella. The amount of fat and cholesterol you'll avoid is astounding, and you'll be pleasantly surprised at how easy and delicious substitutions such as these can be. You'll feel better about how you are treating your body as the cancer-fighting power inside your cells multiplies.

Prostate Cancer

Cancer of the small, walnut-sized prostate gland, located just below the bladder, usually grows very slowly. Next to skin cancer, prostate cancer is the most common cancer in American men and is approximately twice as prevalent in African Americans as in Caucasians. It is the fourth most common cancer among men worldwide, with approximately four hundred thousand new cases diagnosed each year. In fact, many elderly men who die of other diseases often have undiagnosed prostate cancer as well, so incidence is likely much higher than estimates indicate.

The illness is rare among men below age fifty, but incidence increases greatly after this age. To put it in a different perspective, up to 40 percent of eighty-year-old men have prostate cancer.

Prostate cancer incidence is increasing significantly, especially in developed countries. While it's true that doctors are finding more cancers than before due to more frequent screenings and better diagnostic tests, we also seem to be eating ourselves into the disease with high-fat, Western-style diets. As we'll see, dairy products have already been implicated as culprits, and other animal products likely play a role, too, while fruits and vegetables are protective.

Genes may play a small role in a man's risk for developing prostate cancer, so fathers, brothers, and sons of men who have had the disease would be wise to take special care with their diet and lifestyle activities, and to utilize current screening methods as suggested by a doctor. However, all men eventually are at high risk of prostate cancer, so dietary protection is important for everyone. For those at higher risk due to genetics, how we fill our plates can make all the difference in how our genes behave throughout life.

Prostate Protectors

Studies show that fruit and vegetables, especially tomatoes, play a special role in prostate health. A large Harvard study showed that men who ate ten or more servings of tomatoes or tomato products per week had a 35 percent reduction in prostate cancer risk, so don't be shy about taking a few extra tomatoes from the salad bar or having a second helping of marinara sauce on your pasta. Tomatoes and all fruits are naturally high in fiber, with complex and intricate mixtures of vitamins and minerals. But the real credit probably goes to lycopene, the red pigment that gives tomatoes their color. It is a cousin of beta-carotene and an even more powerful antioxidant.

Most people have been enjoying spaghetti with tomato sauce since childhood. Keep up the healthy habit and experiment with "grown-up" versions by adding garlic, onions, peppers, or other delights of the garden. Lycopene is best absorbed when the tomatoes have been cooked, meaning that spaghetti sauce, canned tomatoes, or tomato paste used in soup are all particularly good sources. Even ketchup contains some valuable prostate-protecting benefits, but make sure to add it to veggieburgers or baked potato "fries" (sweet, russet, or new) instead of the usual suspects.

Each time you shop, throw a basket of strawberries in your cart. There's lycopene there, too. You can enjoy them on whole-grain pancakes, in your cereal, or even in a smoothie with bananas, orange juice, blueberries, or any of your other favorite fruits. Add a splash of soy milk for a creamy consistency.

Diets high in vegetables of all shapes, sizes, and colors have proven their worth in decreasing prostate cancer risk, so don't hesitate to try a new variety each week. Try broccolini (small, baby broccoli sprouts) or baby eggplant slices on a homemade pizza. Don't worry, the crust can be bought ready-made and, in just minutes, you'll have a warm, healthy meal. If you're feeling famished, your tomato soup need not be "smooth." Mix in chopped carrots, spinach, corn, beans, or little potato cubes into your bowl of lycopene liquid. Or, if smooth soup is still your favorite, throw a bunch of veggies such as celery, peppers, or squash into the blender and then add the puree for a powerful prostate protector. Add a whole grain roll, and you've taken your vitamins.

The Dangers of Dairy

Several decades ago, when medical research studies began to find serious trouble with dairy products, many people—even some doctors—found it surprising, to say the least. Milk, after all, has been heavily marketed for years. It's even served in school lunch programs. But if we take a moment to look beyond advertising and marketing, we'll be reminded that cow's milk was intended by nature to feed and nourish calves, just as the milk of all mammals was designed to sustain their own offspring. Drinking cow's milk into adulthood could have easily turned out to be nothing more than a peculiar habit, but it has unfortunately led to many serious health problems. Milk drinking has been linked to Type 1 diabetes, breast cancer, overweight, gastrointestinal problems, and prostate cancer.

In 1997, the World Cancer Research Fund and the American Institute for Cancer Research confirmed that separate scientific reviews identified associations between dairy product consumption and prostate cancer risk, and concluded that dairy products should be considered a possible contributor to the development of the disease. By now, more than sixteen studies have shown the link, including two from Harvard University involving large groups of men and using the best research methods available. (For more details, see chapter 2)

As we have seen, dairy products disrupt vitamin D balance, which can lead to prostate cancer. Dairy products also boost blood levels of insulin-like growth factor (IGF-I). Studies in diverse populations have clearly shown that the more IGF-I there is in the blood, the higher your prostate cancer risk. A study of men and women aged fifty-five to eighty-five years showed that the addition of three 8-ounce servings of nonfat or 1 percent milk each day for twelve weeks caused a 10 percent increase in IGF-I. IGF-I levels are significantly lower in people who avoid meat, eggs, and dairy products.

When you skip the dairy aisle and begin selecting protein and calcium sources from plants rather than animals, you'll likely bring your serum IGF-I concentrations back down to a much safer level.

Animal Products: High Fat, No Fiber

Although the problems with dairy products—disrupting vitamin D balance and boosting IGF-I—are seen even with nonfat varieties, the full-fat versions certainly are not any healthier. The high-fat, zero-fiber combination found in most dairy products is likely to increase serum testosterone concentration and activity in men, a dangerous promoter of prostate cancer. If you're hooked on the dairy habit, you are probably getting a good helping of dairy fat throughout the day. Many Western meals douse otherwise healthy vegetables, beans, and grains with greasy cheeses and heavy cream sauces. Try your favorite foods without these and you'll discover a pleasant variety of fresh flavors that have been smothered for too long.

Use Soy Milk Instead

Eliminating cow's milk and other dairy products is an easy way to lower your risk for prostate cancer. But when you *replace* these foods with soy milk and other soy products, you'll also add another measure of defense. In a study of 13,855 Seventh-Day Adventist men, daily soy milk consumption was associated with a 70 percent reduction in prostate cancer risk when compared to those who never drank the beverage. Isoflavones in soy milk have been shown to inhibit the growth of human prostate cancer cells and the enzyme that converts testosterone into a more powerful form of this hormone, called DHT, in the prostate gland. A similar beneficial effect was demonstrated with tofu consumption.

So enjoy your favorite cereals with soy milk. When you pour your morning tea or coffee, simply add soy creamer. Silk brand creamer is a favorite among coffee connoisseurs. Every brand has a unique flavor, so try a few varieties to find the one you like best. They also come with vanilla and chocolate flavorings, in low- and no-fat versions, and with calcium fortification.

Your neighborhood supermarket probably carries an array of soy milks in all flavors, sizes, brands, and consistencies. The same is true for meat "analogs" or alternatives. "NotDogs" and veggieburgers are easy-to-find, tasty alternatives to hot dogs and hamburgers. You'll be amazed to find how many manufacturers tailor products to the meat- and dairy-free consumer.

Risk for prostate cancer clearly increases with consumption of dairy products, saturated fats, and animal fats, and drops with consumption of vegetables, especially tomatoes. By eating a variety of foods from the New Four Food Groups described throughout this book, the risk of prostate cancer will be significantly decreased.

Stopping Cancer after It Starts

Foods not only influence the onset of prostate cancer but also help determine whether it will progress. As we saw in chapter 5, in autopsy studies, cancer cells are found in the prostates of middle-aged and older men surprisingly often. If these cells stay put, they cause no problem. It is only when they begin to multiply and invade neighboring tissues or spread through the bloodstream that serious problems arise. How do we ensure that this doesn't happen? Many prostate cancer researchers are convinced that diet's most important role is not in stopping cancer from starting but in squelching its ability to spread. Happily, the same diet changes that reduce estrogen in women—cutting fat and boosting fiber—do the same to testosterone in men.

Breast Cancer

Breast cancer is the most common cancer among American women and the third most common cancer around the world. It can also occur, albeit rarely, in men. As with prostate cancer, rates are increasing globally, especially in developed countries. And this is where our clues to getting a handle on this illness begin—with environmental factors, especially diet.

A woman's breast consists of glands that produce and secrete milk after the birth of a baby. The breast itself is made up of lobules (glands that make breast milk); ducts (tubes that connect the milk-

A Race for Life

Diagnosed with breast cancer in 1982 at age forty-seven, Ruth Heidrich took drastic steps to conquer her illness. After consulting with physicians who taught her all they knew about breast cancer's relation to diet, she became a strict vegetarian, eating absolutely no animal products. Her diet even avoided food that came in a can, jar, box, or bag.

Feeling the health benefits immediately, she was tempted to try the Ironman Triatholon with its 2.4-mile open ocean swim, 112-mile bike ride, and 26.2-mile marathon. Although it seemed an impossible feat at first, she thought, "What the heck. I have nothing to lose if I'm going to die anyway." That was nearly 20 years ago.

Dr. Heidrich, today a Ph.D. in health administration, has completed numerous Ironman competitions, dozens of marathons, and races from Bangkok to Moscow to the Great Wall of China. She cohosts a weekly talk radio program in Hawaii; lectures on a variety of health, fitness, and nutrition issues; and continues to inspire those who read her books, including *A Race for Life: From Cancer to the Ironman*.

Believing that most health problems and symptoms of aging are the result of eating the wrong foods and not getting enough exercise, Dr. Heidrich has devoted her life to sharing this message so that others can overcome cancer as she has.

producing glands to the nipple); and fatty, connective lymphatic tissue. Most lymphatic vessels of the breast lead to lymph nodes under the arm and are called axillary nodes. Most doctors believe that cancer that has spread to the lymph nodes has a chance of spreading to other organs, making immediate treatment necessary. Modern cancer treatments such as chemotherapy, radiation, and drugs are slowly improving, but we're still attempting to fully understand the disease, especially in regard to preventive measures. However, we've gathered many valuable clues.

Beyond Genetics

We cannot change the genes we're born with, but, luckily they appear to play a minimal role in most cases of breast cancer. About 5 to 10 percent of cases can be blamed on genes passed from either a mother or a father to the next generation. On the other hand, if no one in your family has had cancer, it doesn't mean you are fully protected. Eight in ten women who develop breast cancer do not have a sister or a mother who has had it. With that in mind, it's wise for all women to protect themselves.

Cancer of the breast is usually related to hormones, so all women, regardless of family history, will benefit from keeping hormone levels in check. Hormone preparations commonly given to women after menopause clearly increase the risk, so the nondrug methods for controlling hot flashes and other menopausal symptoms are much preferred. And, as you know by now, diet can have a dramatic effect on hormones. As fatty foods increase the amount of estrogen in the blood, breast cells are stimulated and divide. With every multiplication in cell number, the likelihood that one will turn cancerous increases, but this is easy to alter. By simply eating a low-fat diet of high-fiber vegetables, grains, and other natural plant foods, estrogen levels fall.

Alcohol

After reining in hormones, the next area that deserves prompt attention is alcohol. It doesn't matter whether you have a beer, a martini, or a glass of wine. One alcoholic beverage per day—if it's every day—increases breast cancer risk by roughly 25 percent. The reason, apparently, is that alcohol disrupts the action of the vitamins that protect against cancer, especially folic acid. In fact, studies show that women who drink alcohol can reverse some of their risk by increasing their intake of folic acid, either in supplements or in its natural form in vegetables. However, easing up on alcohol intake is the surest way to reduce risk.

Protecting Yourself with Fruits and Vegetables

Evidence also shows that fruits and vegetables, especially green vegetables, decrease a woman's risk for developing breast cancer. As you know, these foods are packed with protective antioxidants. Every new hue you add to your diet—purple grapes, orange pumpkin, green apples, red beans, brown rice—will shield your cells from inevitable wear, tear, and damage. It doesn't matter how you enjoy them—off the vine, pureed in a shake, or otherwise. The more fruits and vegetables you eat, the lower your breast cancer risk will be. Numerous studies conducted in Poland, Greece, Italy, Canada, Argentina, Japan, Switzerland, and the United States have shown their protective effects. In fact, vegetables and fruits have even been shown to help women beat cancer after diagnosis. One study found that those women who consumed the most fruits and vegetables before going in for breast surgery saw better results afterward. The right diet paired with the right treatment afford cancer patients an important advantage.

More Protection with Exercise

Physical activity also decreases a woman's risk for developing cancer of the breast. With regular exercise, and by consuming and avoiding the above-mentioned foods, a woman will have an easier time maintaining a healthy body weight in childhood and adulthood, which has also been linked to decreasing breast cancer risk.

Colon and Rectal Cancers

Colon and rectal cancers are extremely common, although not everyone knows what these terms actually mean. Here's the anatomy: As we swallow our food, it travels through the esophagus to the stomach, where it is partially broken down, and then moves on to the small intestine, where nutrients are absorbed. (The descriptor "small" refers to this organ's narrow diameter, not its length. With a length of twenty feet, the small intestine is actually the longest portion of the digestive tract.) The small intestine joins the large intestine, or large bowel, which is a strong, muscular tube about five feet long. The first and longest part of the large bowel is called the colon. It absorbs water and mineral nutrients from the food we eat. The rectum is the final six inches of the large intestine.

The fourth most common cancers in the world, colon and rectal cancers have been noted in North America, Europe, and Australia, with more than 60 percent of cases in developed countries. Colon cancer is just as common in men as in women, whereas cancer of the rectum is more prevalent in men. Although colon and rectal cancers differ in the way the cancer develops and progresses, dietary recommendations are similar for both.

Colon cancer is getting a lot more attention these days on morning news programs, in health magazines, and elsewhere. Many lives have been touched, and colon cancer screenings are now being promoted in the way that mammography was as it gained acceptance in routine women's healthcare. Of course, early detection has its value, but let's not forget what it takes to give our bodies a fighting chance of avoiding it altogether.

You may have heard about colorectal cancer beginnings with the formation of polyps, which are tissue growths inside the colon or the rectum. Some polyps are not cancerous, but having polyps does increase your risk of developing colorectal cancer. If a cancer forms in a polyp, it can then grow into the wall of the colon and rectum, where tumor cells eventually break away and spread to other parts of the body.

The cells of the colon aren't so different from cells in the rest of our body. They do their best work with the right tools: generous helpings of fiber in the form of vegetables, whole grains, legumes, and other complex carbohydrates; plenty of exercise throughout life; and avoidance of meat, especially heavily cooked and processed cuts, refined sugars, saturated (animal) fat, eggs, and alcohol.

A Closer Look at Plant Power

Vegetables are strong medicine in the fight against colon cancer. Leafy, green, cruciferous vegetables such as broccoli, cauliflower, Brussels sprouts, and cabbage have been associated with a decreased risk of colon cancer. Research studies following large groups of people over many years have shown reduced colon cancer rates in those consuming the most vegetables and fruits. Part of their value comes from the rich antioxidant content, but they are also loaded with fiber, which, as you know, is like a pipe cleaner for your digestive tract.

One important caveat: Small diet changes are not of much use. Studies comparing people with a bit higher or a bit lower intake of vegetables or other high-fiber foods have not shown much difference. To really help, you need to bring in the vegetables, fruits, and whole grains in a generous way.

Not surprisingly, vegetarians have lower colon cancer rates compared to meat eaters. It's not just that vegetarians' diets are rich in protective vegetables and whole grains. By skipping meats, they skip the carcinogenic chemicals called heterocyclic amines from creatine, amino acids, and natural sugars in meat that form as beef, chicken, or fish are cooked. So give those plant foods all the room they need on your plate. It's time to stop reserving room for just a spoonful of corn or peas. Have a whole meal made of lentils, chickpeas, cauliflower, or spinach, and the wonderful dishes into which they can be transformed. For delightful ideas, look at the recipe section.

Alcohol may play a role in colon cancer, too, just as it does for breast cancer. Even modest amounts—one drink per day or thereabouts—have been shown to increase risk if this becomes part of an ongoing routine. It is not yet clear whether the problem is alcohol's tendency to disrupt the actions of vitamins in the body or a direct effect of alcohol on the body's tender tissues, but the message is clear: Alcohol increases the risk. Intermittent alcohol use does not appear to present this problem.

Ovarian Cancer

Just as most men hadn't thought about their prostate gland until the possibility of it turning cancerous became the talk of the medical community, the same is probably true of women and their ovaries. You can't see them, so they must be healthy and functioning as they should, right? Well, sort of. The health of a woman's ovaries depends on many of the same factors that keep her skin, eyes, bones, and other organs well: her diet, lifestyle habits, and environment. In the case of ovarian cancer, we've had a few surprises. First, the basics.

A woman has two ovaries, one on each side of the pelvis; they are responsible for making eggs and are the main source of the hormones estrogen and progesterone. Although not as widespread as breast cancer, ovarian cancer causes more deaths than any other reproductive organ cancer because it is usually not detected until advanced stages. In fact, most cases of ovarian cancer are found in women over sixty-five. As with any illness, the earlier it is diagnosed, the better the chance that treatments will be effective. If the cancer is found and treated before it has spread outside the ovary, five-year survival is high. However, only about a quarter of ovarian cancers are detected this early, and that's a great reason to put prevention to work today.

Most known risk factors for ovarian cancer relate to hormones. Although most women aren't aware of the amount of hormones in their bodies, they experience their effects in ovulation, pregnancy, breast-feeding, and even premenstrual symptoms. By now you're well aware of how to reduce hormone excesses: Cut the fat and increase the fiber. Or in practical terms, avoid animal products, keep vegetable oils to a minimum, and increase consumption of vegetables, fruits, beans, and grains.

Dairy products may play a special role in ovarian cancer. Daniel Cramer, M.D., of Harvard University, compared the diets of hundreds of women with and without ovarian cancer. Although they were similar in age and other demographic characteristics, the women who developed cancer had had noticeably more dairy products in their diets. The trouble appears to come not just from the animal fats they contain, but from the milk sugar lactose. Lactose must be broken down into two simple sugars—glucose and galactose—during digestion, and galactose appears to be toxic to the ovaries. Compounding the problem, some women have low levels of the enzyme needed to break apart this sugar, allowing galactose to build up. Simply eliminating dairy products in favor of soy milk, rice milk, soy yogurts, or the other delicious nondairy products now on the shelves will eliminate this common source of galactose. As for your calcium requirements, regularly eating cruciferous vegetables, beans, enriched flour, or fortified juices will provide plenty.

Cervical Cancer

We know a good deal about cervical cancer and how to prevent it. Even so, it's important to be vigilant about screenings, as this is an easy and safe measure women can take to minimize their risk. All women should visit their gynecologist every year for an annual exam, which includes a Pap smear. This test reveals abnormal cells that can eventually develop into cancer. Misshapen cells in the cervix can spread to the uterus if not detected early. As it is the second most common cancer in women, there's good reason to catch this problem early.

Human Papilloma Virus

The human papilloma virus (HPV) is extremely common. It exists in a wide variety of forms, most of which are only mild annoyances. But some strains can increase the risk of cervical cancer, and HPV's effect can be detected during a Pap smear as slightly abnormal cells. HPV is passed through skin-to-skin contact during sexual activity. Unfortunately, since condoms don't cover all the skin area, barrier methods can't prevent this disease. The only way to reduce your risk is to limit the number of partners you have or to practice abstinence.

A Surprising Role for Smoking

Cigarettes have been implicated in cervical cancer. In fact, women who smoke are twice as likely to develop the disease as nonsmokers. It may be the increase in free radical damage to cells that is to blame. Of course, we don't need any more evidence to convince us that smoking leads to all sorts of trouble.

Protecting Yourself with Exercise

Surprisingly enough, exercise cuts the risk of cervical cancer. Research studies show that women who are more physically active have a substantially lower incidence of cervical cancer than sedentary women. It may be because active women tend to be leaner. Since body fat produces estrogen, heavier women tend to be at a higher risk for hormone-dependent cancers, including cervical cancer. To lower your risk, simply *get moving*. Try taking daily walks, join a gym, play with a Frisbee, walk with your dog—as long as it gets you moving on a daily basis, you'll strengthen your protection. Start slowly and build up gradually. You may soon find yourself developing a healthy addiction to early-morning jogs or evening aerobics classes.

Vegetables and Fruits Fight Cervical Cancer

Plant foods hold special ingredients—carotenoids, vitamin C, vitamin E—that fight cervical cancer, too. As you'll recall, carotenoids are the dark orange, yellow, and red pigments you see in fruits and vegetables such as tomatoes, carrots, sweet potatoes, and squash. The more of these delicious foods women eat, the lower their risk for cervical cancer. For sufficient vitamin C, reach for citrus fruits (or juices if you're pressed for time) or add peppers, leafy vegetables, or broccoli to your meals. Add strawberries to your oatmeal, whole-grain waffles, or cold cereal. Get your vitamin E by eating whole-grain breads, pasta, or cereal. Nuts are a nice, convenient source, too. By following the New Four Food Groups as described in chapter 3, you'll be sure to get plenty of these nutrients in your body day after day. A diet made up exclusively of these healthy vegetarian foods is low in saturated fat, high in fiber, free of cholesterol, and rich in so many cancer-fighting compounds. Naturally, this is the first step toward cancer prevention.

For the most effective cancer-prevention lifestyle, you'll want to stay away from tobacco products and alcohol, maintain an active lifestyle, and keep excess weight at bay. By sticking to the New Four Food Groups, weight maintenance will be much easier. Each meal you create or select from the vegetable, grain, fruit, or legume group will contain a wide range of cancer-fighting agents. Just as important, a plate filled with healthy plant foods leaves no room for the ones that have been indicted as cancer promoters.

Putting Science to Work

As we have seen, many different forms of cancer are remarkably similar when it comes to prevention. The diet that cuts the risk of prostate cancer probably does the same for breast cancer, colon cancer, cervical cancer, and many other forms. In part this is because some of the protective effects of vegetables and fruits strengthen the immune defenses our bodies use against many illnesses. As scientists continue to explore the range of benefits of these healthful foods, we do not have to wait to put them to work.

8

Treating Yourself to Good Food and Great Health

You've decided to make nutrition a positive force in your life and you're ready to start your journey to vibrant health. Naturally, a travel guide to any destination can be a big help. In this chapter we'll learn how to begin, where to turn at tricky forks along the way, and how to bypass common obstacles on the road to better health. You may have questions already. We'll guide you through some of the challenging terrain you may encounter.

For some children, facing a new food can be a bit of an experience. Just when they feel comfortable eating bright orange carrots, in barges broccoli to disrupt their plate's color scheme. When presented with new foods, most would rather just stick to the foods they already know. Many adults are not so different. It's easy to get stuck in a ham-sandwich rut, like anything we do out of old habit. Some adults, on the other hand, become quite adventurous. They'll read through a recipe, and if it looks like a good bet, they'll pick up the ingredients and try it out.

Your attitudes toward food are worth thinking about, because you're making some big changes now. This is a time for new directions, new traveling companions, and at least a small sense of adventure.

How were vegetables prepared in your family? Were these foods delicately steamed, tender-crisp, and bursting with color? Or just a wilted sidekick to an overcooked steak? Did people enjoy putting meals together, or was it more of a stress? Did your parents often opt for something quick, heavy, and fried? And are they slim, healthy, and active today? Preparing healthy food can be a most satisfying experience. With a few tips, your time in the kitchen can become a pleasure.

Making Friends with Healing Foods

When making any life changes, it is not a bad idea to seek out others with similar goals. Here's where cooking classes are a big help. Find one at local health clinics, community centers, or vegetarian associations. You'll find a world of new flavors and get a lot of your questions answered, too. Having a chance to try new foods makes a big difference. You'll be much more interested in healthy new foods when you know tasty ways to use them. You're sure to find the dishes that will become regulars on your menu.

Preparing food together can be a lovely way to spend an evening or an afternoon, and you may soon find your family members experimenting along with you—especially young children. If not, grab a friend who might be interested in getting together each week for the simple joy of trying new recipes and enjoying food.

If you are going through cancer treatment, your time in the kitchen may be scarce. Here's where friends or relatives can step in. Although others would *like* to assist you, they're often not sure what to do. If treatments make you tired, ask them to prepare blender drinks or soups to suit your taste. They can stock your freezer with individual portion packages to carry you through the week. The people who care about you will be delighted to do something that really helps.

When you'd like a soothing comfort food, you'll find excellent choices from the recipe section of this book: Warm Oatmeal, Mashed Potatoes, Neat Loaf, Tomato Soup (served with fresh, whole grain bread), Blueberry Muffins, and Apricot Smoothie. These are even more comforting when you know they're made with wholesome, nourishing ingredients.

Keeping It Simple

Some people equate healthy eating with spending hours at the stove cooking beans from scratch, or having to grow their own vegetable garden. They may also assume that complicated combinations of food must be eaten at each meal. Actually, none of this is necessary.

Simplicity can be yours, even on the best diet possible. Your basic lunch or dinner can be easy to assemble yet highly nutritious.

- First, have salad ready or steam some vegetables. Perhaps you enjoy salads when they're beautifully arranged and placed in front of you. Yet when you rush in the door hungry, the last thing you want to do is wash greens. Here's a solution: Pick up one or two very large Tupperware-type containers. Tightly sealed, they will keep salad fresh for up to four days. Mix up a huge salad once or twice a week. Do your salad-making in the company of another person, music, or a favorite radio program. Rinse and chop all sorts of colorful veggies: romaine lettuce, carrots, cucumbers, squash, finely sliced red cabbage or kale, colored peppers, and even cauliflower or broccoli. (Don't add dressing or tomatoes; these will make everything soggy.) Cut up raw vegetable sticks while you're at it, or just buy them cleaned and cut, and keep them in a bowl or a plastic bag near the front of the fridge. Sliced raw carrots, celery, peppers, cauliflower, and zucchini are a great snack for the car or while you're reading or watching TV. Bags of prewashed salad mix can be purchased and stored it in the same way. To increase the cancer-fighting power of salad mixes, add red, orange, and yellow vegetables. In the recipe section you'll find several nutritious dressings, such as the Liquid Gold Dressing on page 176. These can be used on the salad, baked potato, or on steamed vegetables.
- Add something starchy, like rice or baked potatoes. Make brown rice in batches that will last for several meals. Rice can be quickly warmed in a steamer or a microwave a day or two later.

Millet and quinoa (a South American grain) are even faster to cook than brown rice; they're ready in twenty minutes.

You'd hesitate to turn the oven on for one potato, but if you bake half a dozen potatoes and yams at once, they can be used at future meals. (While you're at it, make Roasted Red Peppers, page 206.)

- Complete your meal with a veggieburger or marinated tofu. Or toss some chickpeas or other beans on your salad. The range of soy foods now available at supermarkets is immense. In quality and variety they've come a long way in the past six years. Look at new soy products in the deli, produce, refrigerator, freezer, and packaged foods sections. There are burgers, beverages, instant mixes, marinated tofu, tempeh in sauces, and frozen soybeans in a pod (edamame). These make food preparation as simple or as elaborate as you could wish. The new, very-low-fat veggie "meats" and "poultry" can be used in just about any of your old recipes.

If speed and convenience have tied you to take-out, you'll see that there is a vast array of healthy meals out there. Quick vegan meals at home are easy with the right recipe. Of course, you can always stick with take-out restaurants serving meatless meals. Thai, Chinese, and Italian are easy options.

A Helpful Hint

"I made blender drinks using three basic ingredients: fruit; tofu or soy yogurt; and nuts (walnuts, almonds, or cashews). I liked it to taste different each day, and I'd vary the fruit or nuts used. Sometimes I'd add a little cinnamon or nutmeg. This would be a quick source of nutrition at home. I also kept individual portions in the freezer. Then, when I had to go somewhere for the day, I'd take one or two portions along, letting them thaw on the way. As I got better at it, I realized I could use the same basic idea with pureed vegetables, ending up with a creamy soup."

J. S., VANCOUVER, BRITISH COLUMBIA

Raw vs. Cooked

Are raw vegetables and fruits more protective than cooked? Sometimes yes, but not in every instance. A diet of raw vegetables and fruits, plus sprouted seeds, nuts, and grains, is very rich in vitamins C, E, other antioxidants, and fiber. Scandinavian research has shown this diet to reduce certain toxic substances in the colon, including those substances related to cancer risk. People with rheumatoid arthritis also have reported decreased pain, swelling, and stiffness using this diet. Loading up on fresh raw produce, especially items at their seasonal peak, will always invigorate your cells, but cooking has advantages, too.

Some people may find that cooked foods are easier to chew and digest. You may not have realized that cooking makes it easier to absorb some antioxidants. (Chewing well helps, too.) For example, you'll get 33 percent more beta-carotene from cooked, pureed carrots than from raw carrots because the heat breaks the plant cells open, making some protective substances more readily available. Cooking also increases absorption of lycopene from tomatoes. And, while you're making your next meal, remember this: Some cell-nourishing substances actually form during cooking. Whereas raw garlic contains dozens of protective compounds, even more are created when you mince the cloves and then simmer them in your pasta sauce. The same is true for dozens of other plant foods. When eaten with the peel (as with carrots or baked potatoes), the amount of antioxidants and fiber is considerably higher than when the peel is removed. (Use organic produce to avoid pesticides in the peel.)

Research on foods and cancer risk involves millions of people eating just about every vegetable and fruit you can think of, prepared in more ways than you can imagine. But findings can be summarized very simply: Whether they are raw, cooked, yellow, red, orange, white, purple, blue, or green, vegetables and fruits *protect*. Let vegetables, fruits, and whole grains be the foundation of every meal, and their protective substances will work around the clock.

Cruciferous vegetables such as broccoli, cauliflower, and cabbage are hard to digest raw. A bit of cooking helps enormously. If you have intestinal problems, you may need to limit raw foods for a time, because the fiber may be physically irritating. In this case use juices, and vegetables and fruits that are cooked. And stock up on individual portion packs of low-sodium tomato or tomato-vegetable juices. These are handy to pop in your bag when you go away from home.

Does Tea or Coffee Affect Cancer Risk?

Asia has given us a healthy appetite for many vegetable, rice, and tofu delicacies. Now green tea is gaining popularity as well. Research from Asia suggests that regular use of green tea contributes to low cancer rates. Women who drink four cups or more each day have breast cancer rates that are 25 percent lower than others. Regular tea drinkers are less likely to have certain cancers of the digestive system. Tea's protective effects seem to be due to antioxidants and to its ability to inactivate carcinogens, stop out-of-control cell growth, and support the natural death of defective cells. The protective compounds are present in the green and black variety, whether it's loose or in tea bags, decaffeinated or regular, and allowed to steep for a short or a long time. Green and black teas come from the same Asian plant *(Camellia sinensis),* the main difference being that black tea is roasted at low temperatures for a long period, resulting in a darker leaf color and a more intense flavor and aroma. Both types of tea seem to have similar biological effects. When black tea is loaded with cream, milk, sugar, or artificial sweeteners, however, it may be doing more harm than good.

Roasted coffee beans do not have these antioxidant actions, though the message about coffee and cancer risk is not clear. Several studies suggest that coffee may affect DNA and increase risk of bladder and ovarian cancers. Extremely hot drinks can have a physically damaging effect on cells in the mouth and throat, making them more vulnerable to cancer if used repeatedly.

Food Safety and Food Storage

From parts of the world that have little refrigeration available, we have learned that some forms of cancer are caused by food that has gone bad. Throw out moldy food. Store whole grains and legumes in dry conditions, for example, in glass jars or plastic buckets. Nuts and seeds such as whole flaxseeds come with protective packaging provided by nature; they can be stored in dry conditions without refrigeration. Keep unshelled nuts in a cool, dry place, preferably the freezer or the refrigerator. Refrigerate perishable foods.

When oxidized, omega-3 fatty acids can develop a rancid, fishy smell. (Fish oils also have omega 3s, which is why fish can have the same smell.) When oxidized (rancid), omega-3s may not be a nutritional benefit; in fact, they can be harmful. In practical terms this means that you should keep flax oil and ground flaxseed in the freezer or the refrigerator. Flaxseed should be ground freshly before use, or it may be stored in the freezer for several months. Keep wheat germ in the refrigerator or the freezer, too.

Make sure to wash your fruits and vegetables. They do not normally harbor disease-causing bacteria. However, produce can be tainted by animal manure that was used as fertilizer, or contaminated by poor hand-washing.

During cancer treatments, your natural defenses are likely to be weaker, so take extra care against foodborne illness. Use juices that are freshly squeezed or pasteurized. Steer clear of meat, poultry, and eggs, and salads made with mayonnaise, as they often harbor bacteria that can lead to food poisoning.

Meals on the Go

More than a quarter of the meals eaten by North Americans are eaten away from home. Though meals served in a typical American household are high in fat (32 percent of calories) and low in fiber, restaurant meals can be even worse, unless you know where to look. When you travel for work, visit loved ones, or attend out-of-town medical treatments, healthy food can seem miles away from the highway or the airport. Luckily, there are folks who have come to the rescue.

The Vegetarian Journal's Guide to Natural Foods Restaurants in the U.S. and Canada (Wayne, N.J.: Avery Publishing Group) is published every few years. This guide is great to keep in the car or in your suitcase. It features more than two thousand restaurants, juice bars, and delicatessens with healthy selections. Two Web sites (www.vegdining.com and www.vegeats.com/restaurants) give guidance about restaurants. Click on the city you're going to, or where you live, and you'll find a list of local eating spots, with a description of each. A little preparation takes one travel worry away, not to mention the enjoyment you'll get out of sampling a nice variety of regional vegetarian fare.

Whether you're in an airport, some exotic destination, or close to home, ethnic restaurants prepare out-of-this-world creations with tofu and beans.

Most airlines these days can be very accommodating to passengers who request healthy meals. United Airlines, for example, serves half a million vegetarian meals every year. When you book a flight, request a nondairy vegetarian meal. Still, you may prefer a homemade favorite packed in a container with a tight-fitting, spill-proof lid.

Three take-along foods that can help you assemble a meal anywhere include:

1. protein-rich foods such as marinated tofu, hummus, or soup
2. fortified soy milk or rice milk
3. a little salad dressing for vegetables

With these three items in hand, a tasty meal comes together easily. For breakfast, dry cereal, oatmeal, and fruit are widely available. You can use your soy milk on cereal or in tea. For lunch and supper, baked potatoes, salads, rice, pasta, and vegetables can be found in airports, planes, trains, and bus depots. Use your dressing on the baked potato, rice, or salad, and complete the meal with the protein-rich food you brought. Salsa also works as a low-fat dressing or potato topping and can be found at many food outlets. For meals or snacks you can also purchase fruit or juices. While undergoing cancer treatments, good foods to bring are a blended soup or smoothie.

Social Events

Special occasions often revolve around exactly those foods that trigger and promote cancer. But a healthy diet certainly doesn't mean an end to your social life. On the next pages we'll consider two food-related events and present some options. See what would be the best choice for you.

Eating in Company

You're invited to a barbecue, complete with slabs of meat on the grill, fried chicken, and a keg of beer. Does the menu include foods you'd be comfortable eating? You could:

1. Turn down the invitation.
2. Show up; eat and drink everything that's served.
3. Offer to bring along one of your own favorite (healthy) dishes, or see if the host suggests alternatives.

Here's how each of these options might turn out.

1. *Turn down the invitation.* You could have a relaxing evening on your own or in other company. You won't be tempted by foods you don't want, nor will you feel like a party pooper. It's possible that in adopting healthier habits, you are moving away from some of the friends or work associates attending this event. Possibly you'll see them less often, at least not at this sort of occasion. For some people, however, this isn't the ideal choice. Even though everyone at the barbecue doesn't share your values about health, the group may include warm, caring people with whom you want to strengthen bonds, not create separation.

2. *Show up; eat and drink everything that's served.* After all, it's just for this one evening, and cancer isn't caused by one incident. At least this way, you don't stick out like a sore thumb. Yet this choice may leave you feeling that you weren't true to yourself. Since many social events revolve around unhealthy foods and beverages, sooner or later you'll need to figure out how to include options that are more supportive to you.

3. *Offer to bring along one of your own favorite (healthy) dishes, or see if the host suggests alternatives.* At a company barbecue, or if your host can easily include alternatives, he or she may be delighted to add a few items to the menu. Practical suggestions may be welcome, such as bean salads, veggie "meats," whole grain rolls, tomato juice, or fruits. In other situations it will be much simpler if you bring a few items. You could pick up something from a natural foods deli, or from the cooler at a local supermarket: marinated tofu, hummus and crackers, vegetarian nori rolls, or other healthy convenience foods. You might

prepare Zucchini Pockets or Salsa Fresca (see pages 163 and 174), and add a gorgeous assortment of sliced raw veggies or a variety of flavored veggieburgers with all the toppings (lettuce, tomato, onions, soy cheese, or maybe grilled Portobello mushrooms).

Either way, you'll support your new conviction that healthy eating can be festive. People love delicious food; even if it happens to be good for them. Since so many people are cutting back on meat and taking an interest in health, you can be certain that these foods will be a hit with other partygoers, too.

Family Matters

Sometimes dinnertime at family gatherings can be a bit stressful, especially when change is in the air. Food is a focal point, and the table is always loaded. Your aunts try to outdo each other with rich dishes. Though some of your relatives may have major health problems, it hasn't occurred to anyone to lighten up the menu. You'd like to start eating a different way. You should:

1. Tell them how bad this food is for them.
2. Begin new food traditions by adding tasty, attractive vegetarian dishes you know they'll love.
3. Start new activities that aren't entirely focused on food.

Here are some ways these choices might turn out.

1. *Tell them how bad this food is for them.* Some people may listen to you, while others will see it as a guilt trip. Though they become uncomfortable, they probably won't respond by giving up the heavy food. If you're going to discuss the health value of the foods offered, the time to do it is in the menu-planning stage, not after everything has been prepared.

2. *Begin new food traditions by adding tasty, attractive vegetarian dishes you know they'll love.* Socializing around heavy, fatty meals is a ritual that originated long ago, when people's everyday food was considerably lower in fat, and often meager. Though times have changed, the idea that celebration equals rich food persists.

Yet people are open to change. If you arrive with food

contributions that are attractive, tasty, and healthy, these may get an enthusiastic reception. No one will mind. In fact, these may become an essential part of future gatherings. You're likely to attract a following, and you'll have something good to eat. Try Eggplant Manicotti, Barbecue-style Portobello, Thai Wrap, Stuffed Winter Squash, Holiday Fruitcake, or Cranberry Apple Tea.

3. *Start new activities that aren't entirely focused on food.* On your own, or with the help of a few family members, shift the focus to doing things, instead of simply eating. Here are a few new traditions that some families have come up with, adapted to suit the very young and the elderly. In the autumn, take a gentle stroll through a nearby park or along a lake to see the leaves turn. If everyone can manage, go for a more strenuous forest hike. With colder weather, some families celebrate with a skating party. When it's warmer they play ball or croquet. If the gathering must be indoors, there are still numerous possibilities: board games, table hockey, pool, darts, or bowling. Such events can include a meal or snacks, after everyone has worked up an appetite. But it needn't be an immense feast that leaves people stuffed to the brim.

As you begin to change your diet, you are not alone. Everywhere, people are lightening up the menu to trim their waistline, cut cholesterol, or just feel better. With these simple tips, you can enjoy your new journey in good company.

9

Fitness, Friendship, and Freedom from Stress

Three vital lifestyle ingredients, beyond diet, help to keep you in vibrant health and make life worth living. These are exercise, stress reduction, and your interconnection with other people. Each plays a part in preventing disease; each is of primary importance to cancer survivors. This chapter shows how they help and gives practical tips for building them into your life.

Is exercise a part of your life, or has it managed to slip away? For many of us, life has become more sedentary than ever. And if you've gained a bit of weight or if you're not well, exercise can be a daunting prospect.

We have similar problems when it comes to stress. Sometimes the subtlest aggravations throughout your day can add up considerably over time. Do you enjoy a brisk thirty-minute walk during your lunch hour, or do you race around town, running errands in the bustling traffic? Do you make stress-free dates with people you really enjoy, eating out, trying a new exercise class, or just having a good conversation? Or have all of your encounters with people diminished to hectic meetings and hasty required rituals? It's always a good idea to take stock of where the hours of your day are going. Sometimes it takes a little readjustment—renewing friend-

Powerful Medicine

"If the effects of exercise could be bottled, it would be the most widely prescribed medication."

LINN GOLDBERG, M.D.

ships, making time for small indulgences—to realize how many gratifying activities have slipped away.

Believe it or not, exercise, stress reduction, and personal relationships can play important roles in boosting health (for cancer survivors, too). Now is the time to look at whether you are getting all you can from these areas of life.

The Research: Good Reason to Move

Exercise is a vital way to send extra pounds packing and to lower your risk for cancer. It also lowers blood pressure and cholesterol, and it improves your circulation, your sleep, your sex life, your social life, and your frame of mind. In the long run it reduces risk of heart disease, diabetes, osteoporosis, arthritis, and obesity.

Its effectiveness has been most clearly demonstrated against colon cancer. One major study looked at cancer rates among seventeen thousand male alumni from Harvard University. Those who burned 2,500 calories a week cut their risk of colon cancer in *half*. No, they didn't spend hours in the weight room or running around a track. This activity level is the equivalent of a brisk, one-hour walk every day, plus an extra hour of gardening or golf during the week.

Another study, done in Utah and Minnesota, showed that people whose weekly activity amounted to at least 700 calories (equal to just three hours of walking) reduced their colon cancer risk by 40 percent. The benefits of regular exercise in preventing colon cancer have been confirmed by more than twenty studies, involving several million people, in North America, Europe, Asia, and Australia. Vigorous physical exercise throughout life is best. But starting a fitness program at any age seems to help.

Exercise offers some protection against prostate cancer, too, but it seems to require working up more of a sweat. In the Harvard study, men whose activity levels amounted to at least 4,000 calories per week cut their risk of prostate cancer, compared to men who were inactive. Over the course of a week this is the equivalent of five hours of jogging, squash, racquetball, energetic tennis, mountain backpacking, or skiing. A protective effect against lung cancer was shown, too, in 40 percent less lung cancer among those exercising enough to burn 3,000 calories per week.

A California study showed that young women who get about four hours of exercise a week have 40 percent less risk of developing breast cancer. Research in Sweden showed that women who worked at sedentary jobs and didn't exercise in their leisure time were three times more likely to develop breast cancer compared to more active women. Similarly, other research found that women doing the least amount of physical activity were four times more likely to get endometrial cancer. Moderate, regular exercise seems to reduce risk of cervical and ovarian cancers, too.

After reviewing the considerable research linking exercise and cancer prevention, the American Institute of Cancer Research and the World Cancer Research Fund recommend that people with sedentary occupations take an hour's brisk walk, or similar exercise, daily, and also exercise vigorously for at least one extra hour per week.

How Does Exercise Decrease Cancer Risk?

People who exercise regularly are more likely to practice other healthful habits, such as consuming less meat, other fatty foods, and alcohol; avoiding tobacco; eating more vegetables and other plant foods; and managing their weight. Yet beyond these, it seems that physical activity contributes directly to decreased cancer risk. Exercise is an excellent jump start on a journey to better health. Here are even more surprising benefits of an active lifestyle:

1. When we exercise, food passes more quickly through the intestine. As a result, substances in food that promote cancer contact the intestinal wall for a shorter time and are less likely to be absorbed or otherwise damage cells.
2. Physical activity improves the way the body uses insulin, giving less support for out-of-control cell growth.

3. Exercise decreases estrogen production in women. This reduces risk of breast cancer and other hormone-related cancers.
4. Exercise may boost immune strength by increasing the number of white blood cells called natural killer cells in your bloodstream. These cells lock onto cancer cells and eliminate them. Researchers at Loma Linda University in California found that brisk walking (forty-five minutes, five times a week, over the course of fifteen weeks) increased natural killer cell activity.
5. Keeping fit may also improve your body's ability to produce other cancer-fighting immune cells: T cells and B cells, which make antibodies that can attack and destroy invading viruses or bacteria, as well as interleukin-1, a substance that helps white blood cells function more effectively.

The More Exercise, the Better? Yes—to a Point

This doesn't mean you have to take up marathons. While an hour of daily activity really does power up the immune system, exercising to the point of exhaustion can have the opposite effect. After a three-hour run, trained marathon runners showed less natural killer cell activity for twenty-one hours. This amount of intense exercise can be a stressor. So when it comes to exercise, more is not always better.

Exercise during and after Cancer Treatment

Exercise is good for cancer patients, too. Those who are physically active while going through treatment feel better, sleep better, have less fatigue, and report a better quality of life. They may also tolerate treatments better and recover faster after surgery, radiation, or chemotherapy. Overall, they are stronger. With as little as four days of inactivity, your muscles lose strength and start shrinking. Since exercise increases the amounts of the "feel good" brain proteins known as endorphins, it is a natural mood elevator. This is as true for cancer patients as it is for people who are well. A group of women with breast cancer who were going through chemotherapy in Seattle did a home-based exercise program. They found that those who exercised had fewer "bad days" (when they were very tired) and more "good days," with very little fatigue.

Of course, you need to check with your physician before beginning any exercise program. It is important to be sensitive to your need for rest, yet not be put off exercise because of fatigue, which can sometimes be a fine line. Fatigue is common among cancer patients, especially if they're receiving chemotherapy or radiation treatments. As your body needs your energy for healing, don't increase your stress by overdoing exercise. You'll find your comfort zone. A British study found that every one of the advanced cancer patients in the program was able to increase his or her activity level without adding to their fatigue. With exercise, quality of life increased and anxiety decreased. In fact, those with most fatigue when they started experienced the best results.

For those in treatment or who are healing from cancer, exercise can mean gentle movements along with music, an exercise video, or a TV program. It can mean lifting 3- to 5-pound weights. Some people find that joining a group is the best way to make sure they to get out and exercise regularly. If you get stuck, a physiotherapist can help you create a program personalized for your needs.

Planning Your Exercise Program

A fitness program should combine activities that stretch and strengthen muscles and increase endurance. A few stretches or yoga poses are a great way to begin. Strength building can come from workouts at the gym several times a week, or from equivalent activities such as gardening.

For most people, walking is an ideal way to maintain health and fitness. The faster your walking pace, the better. If you have not been exercising regularly, let your speed increase gradually instead of leaping into a high-intensity program. Find an area where you will enjoy your surroundings, such as a park, a beach, or a quiet road.

Use comfortable walking shoes. For ease of movement, your walking shoe should be light, have a low heel, a sole thick enough to cushion the foot on gravel roads, and plenty of flexibility in the forefoot. Running shoes, designed to absorb the shock of running, and reduce injuries, are usually too rigid for walking. They have higher heels, which interfere with the natural motion of the foot.

To begin a regular walking practice, walk at a comfortable pace, slightly above a stroll. Set a goal of twenty to thirty minutes at this speed each day, increasing gradually. How fast you progress is entirely up to you. Don't emphasize speed so much that you miss out on enjoyment. Go for an invigorating walk after dinner instead of retreating to the sofa. Especially in warmer months, you may find you want to stay out longer and longer. There is nothing like the changing scenery of trees, neighborhoods, and even busy people to put you in a new state of mind.

If you have associated exercise with jogging along a smoggy roadway at 6:00 A.M., or pedaling on a stationary bike for as long as boredom will allow, discard those miserable connections for good. Physical activity that adds stress isn't what you're after. The real goal is to find enjoyable ways of moving, so you'll continue to do it every day. Of course, many people enjoy jogging, running, weight lifting, and structured aerobics. But these are just a few of the possibilities.

Our bodies are designed to walk, dance, cycle, participate in games, and play with children. These activities can get your heart pumping and get you moving. We do them for fun, and we burn calories in the process. If you put on music and start dancing in the living room, your dog will likely be very pleased to join in (or at least enjoy the show). Maybe your next-door neighbor would, too. Community centers have many creative programs and classes that involve dance, yoga, and many other types of movement. Buy a volleyball net, Ping-Pong table, basketball hoop, kite, toboggan, soccer ball, or Frisbee and play with your children, grandchildren, or neighbors of all ages. Climb a hill near your home every day. Walk around the neighborhood and smell the roses. Pick a path that is rich with sights, sounds, and smells. One of the best ways to develop a friendship is by meeting regularly for power walks together.

You'll tone up all muscle groups by combining different forms of exercise. Here are a few activities, along with the calories used in an hour by a person weighing 135 pounds and by one weighing 165 pounds.

An enjoyable workout doesn't end as you leave the gym. Its feel-good effects often permeate a handful of other habits. As your body begins to change, energy rises, and your mind destresses, meat, alcohol, and tobacco often lose their appeal. Loading up on healthful plant foods works so well for weight loss that your desire for fatty foods dwindles.

CALORIES USED IN AN HOUR

ACTIVITY (MODERATE ACTIVITY LEVEL UNLESS STATED)	CALORIES USED BY 135-POUND PERSON	CALORIES USED BY 165-POUND PERSON
Aerobics	459	561
Badminton	367	449
Bed exercise	122	150
Bowling, easy level	122	150
Canoeing, rowing	337	412
Cycling, slow	184	225
Cycling 15 mph	398	486
Dancing, recreational	367	449
Gardening	306	374
Golf with hand cart	245	299
Hiking	306	374
Jogging 6 mph	625	763
Playing piano	153	187
Skating	398	486
Squash or racquetball	612	748
Step aerobics	698	853
Stretching	122	150
Swimming	367	449
Table tennis	245	299
Walking 2 mph	147	180
Walking 4 mph	259	317
Walking 5 mph	478	584

Weight Management

The combination of exercise and a low-fat, plant-based diet will help keep your weight at a healthy level. That's important because being overweight definitely raises risk of endometrial cancer, and it probably also increases the likelihood of breast, colon, kidney, and other cancers.

To find out what is a healthy weight for you, check your body mass index, or BMI. The American Institute of Cancer Research and the World Cancer Research Fund recommend keeping your BMI between 18.5 and 25, and limiting weight gain during adulthood to 11 pounds.

To find your BMI, locate your height in inches along the top line of the following table. Then, in the column at the left, find your weight in pounds. Where that column and row intersect is your BMI. A healthy BMI is in the shaded area, between 18.5 and 25.

If your BMI is above 25, here are four keys to bringing your weight down:

1. Build exercise into your life, with a future goal of an hour every day, plus an extra hour of vigorous activity at least once a week.
2. Make health a top goal in your life.
3. Center your diet on whole plant foods, with about 15 percent of your calories from fat. Make your portions reasonable and avoid rushed meals.
4. Eat when you're hungry; don't eat when you're not. It is very tempting to eat when you're bored, tired, upset, or stressed. Yet food doesn't really solve the problems of boredom, fatigue, emotional upset, or stress. Finding real solutions may mean that you need to make other changes in your life.

Stress Management

We all know that our thoughts can affect our body. Who hasn't felt his or her heartbeat race or internal butterflies take flight just as a critical event unfolds? As proof of this, who hasn't had an embarrassing thought and then blushed? We now have evidence that

Body Mass Index

Weight (in pounds)	Height (inches)												
	60	61	62	63	64	65	66	67	68	69	70	71	72
100	20	19	18	18	17	17	16	16	15	15	14	14	14
105	21	20	19	19	18	17	17	16	16	16	15	15	14
110	21	21	20	19	19	18	18	17	17	16	16	15	15
115	22	22	21	20	20	19	19	18	17	17	17	16	16
120	23	23	22	21	21	20	19	19	18	18	17	17	16
125	24	24	23	22	21	21	20	20	19	18	18	17	17
130	25	25	24	23	22	22	21	20	20	19	19	18	18
135	26	26	25	24	23	22	22	21	21	20	19	19	18
140	27	26	26	25	24	23	23	22	21	21	20	20	19
145	28	27	27	26	25	24	23	23	22	21	21	20	20
150	29	28	27	27	26	25	24	23	23	22	22	21	20
155	30	29	28	27	27	26	25	24	24	23	22	22	21
160	31	30	29	28	27	27	26	25	24	24	23	22	22
165	32	31	30	29	28	27	27	26	25	24	24	23	22
170	33	32	31	30	29	28	27	27	26	25	24	24	23
175	34	33	32	31	30	29	28	27	27	26	25	24	24
180	35	34	33	32	31	30	29	28	27	27	26	25	24
185	36	35	34	33	32	31	30	29	28	27	27	26	25
190	37	36	35	34	33	32	31	30	29	28	27	26	26
195	38	37	36	35	34	33	32	31	31	30	29	28	27
200	39	38	37	35	34	33	32	31	30	30	29	28	27
205	40	39	37	36	35	34	33	32	31	30	29	29	28
210	41	40	38	37	36	35	34	33	32	31	30	29	28
215	42	41	39	38	37	36	35	34	33	32	31	30	29
220	43	42	40	39	38	37	36	35	34	33	32	31	30

stress, and how you respond to it, can alter your body's resistance to cancer. And it can certainly change your quality of life.

As you'll recall from chapter 5, your immune system uses specialized white blood cells, known as T cells, to seek out unusual cells that shouldn't be there. Some white blood cells even produce anticancer chemicals, much like those used in chemotherapy, except they don't harm healthy cells. And natural killer cells head for tiny tumors and devour the diseased tissues. As a result, many tumors never make it beyond the early stages.

Stress affects cancer risk because your immune system functions differently when you are under stress. When you sense a threat (even one that is imaginary), your body gets ready to defend itself. Your heart races, blood pressure builds, and muscles tense to prepare for swift, powerful action. In primitive times, these changes helped our ancestors deal with dangerous situations such as sudden storms, falling trees, or physical attacks. In the stresses we face nowadays, these responses are often not appropriate. You don't need tight muscles and a rapid heart rate when you resolve a business dispute, face a conflict at home, or deal with a traffic jam. But old habits are hard to break. With modern-day stress, mental clarity, good communication skills, and a sense of humor are likely to be of much greater value.

When you are stressed, your programmed physical response is to temporarily disable your immune system and get ready for fight or flight. You turn off your inner surveillance and prepare to defend yourself in a different way, from the danger outside your body. The brain signals the adrenal glands to produce hormones (such as cortisol) that inhibit the immune system. These hormones are like synthetic corticosteroid drugs. Corticosteroids are so good at suppressing the immune system that they are used to disable the immune system's response to allergic conditions, skin grafts, and organ transplants. Thus, having large amounts of stress-related hormones in your system means you have let down your guard against cancer. Constant stress can make it easier for cancer to spread.

Stress-related emotions that may reduce resistance to cancer include these: repressed anger, a feeling of helplessness, hopelessness, depression, and grief. Not surprisingly, certain cancers have proven to be more likely after stressful life events. Researchers have found, for example, that the risk of developing breast cancer is higher after a woman has lost a spouse or a close friend. This intensity is reflected in changes in the immune system. Australian researchers observed changes in T-cell function in twenty-six people who had recently lost a spouse, finding them significantly lower than for people who were not mourning a loved one. Depressed T-cell activity has been shown in women who had lost their jobs. Natural killer cell activity is also lower in individuals under stress.

Stressful experiences can influence the likelihood of contracting the skin cancer known as melanoma. Researchers at Yale University looked at the lives of fifty-six people with melanoma, and a similar group without skin cancer. The melanoma patients had experienced significantly more divorces, marital separations, deaths of a spouse or family member, bankruptcies, and unemployment during the five years before diagnosis.

Successfully Handling Stress

It is not the events themselves that cause stress reactions, but how you respond to them. Everyone does not handle a particular situation in the same way.

For several decades, psychologists have been trying to figure out whether personality type plays a role in the development of cancer. Though the picture is far from clear, a few clues have emerged. Two characteristics seem common among women with breast cancer: avoidance of conflict, and denial of feelings. When these two characteristics are combined with stressful life events such as separation and loss, they may contribute to the likelihood of breast cancer. Of course, many people who have difficulty expressing emotion will never develop cancer, but learning to deal with and air a range of feelings is good for all of us, lowering risk of disease being just one of many benefits.

Over the years, various studies have shown that women who show a "fighting spirit"—a combative attitude toward their breast cancer—have less recurrence and longer survival compared to those who respond with passivity and helplessness. This doesn't mean that those with the "fighting spirit" were angry all the time, though they were sometimes. These women accepted and expressed their feelings, and they took active measures to relieve anger and frustration.

A small Massachusetts study of five-year breast cancer survivors gave some hints as to a survivor personality. What helped these women cope with cancer was their work, their families, some sort of spiritual dimension in their lives, and the information they gathered to help them regain health. Their vulnerability during the experience led to profound changes in how they viewed life and how they lived it. Though they had some fear of a recurrence, they described positive aspects of their cancer experiences, and were clear that they had gained something from them.

One West Coast woman summarized one of the profound lessons she had learned during the year when she overcame a nasopharyngeal cancer. "I can now go to a mental state that makes practically anything okay. I can calm myself with my thoughts. It took me quite a while to learn this. When I was first diagnosed, and during the early stages of treatment, I used tapes from the cancer center. Now I don't have to take the outside world's view of things, or anyone else's view of things. Just because it's supposed to be stressful doesn't mean it has to be that way for me."

Increasing Skills

There's a big difference between denying your feelings, and allowing yourself to fully experience and accept your feelings. This is one of the lessons to be learned through meditation, relaxation techniques, or sometimes through a support group or spiritual practices.

Both relaxation and meditation are techniques that show great promise as tools for creating health in the body. Research has provided biochemical evidence that by meditating, the harmful effects of stress can be reduced, for example, by dropping corticosteroid levels. Meditators also can increase their levels of substances that may be beneficial, such as melatonin. This is news in the West, although yogic practitioners in India have used these tools for thousands of years. Meditation and relaxation techniques can reduce the anxiety and helplessness that often accompany cancer. This can make it easier to come to decisions about treatment. When you relax the body by either method, you support your body's anticancer defenses.

Meditation

Meditation usually takes place in a sitting position with the eyes closed. (It can be done lying down, but if you fall asleep you won't be meditating anymore.) A common technique is to let your attention sweep through your body, moving wherever it is drawn, also noticing thoughts and feelings. The idea is not to suppress, analyze,

Choosing an Attitude

In *How to Live between Office Visits* (HarperCollins audiotape), surgeon Bernie Siegel says, "I learned many years ago that when I meet a genuinely happy person, it is not because they have had only good fortune. I know they are choosing their attitude." Through his books and audiotapes, Dr. Siegel's words give comfort, hope, and peace of mind to millions. "Disease isn't punishment, it is a part of life. If you are going to accept the gift of life, you are going to accept its difficulties." You can accept difficulties, and through them learn and grow.

or judge your thoughts and feelings, even those that seem negative or disturbing. One simply notices the thoughts and feelings, then gently lets them go. Like waves breaking at the shore, you can't be sure what will flow in, but you can be sure it will easily flow back out. Avoid the temptation to pursue thoughts and ideas that arrive. Consciously let your mind drift.

It is especially helpful to use a particular focus, such as your breathing. The purpose of the focus is to "anchor" the mind when it becomes too busy or distracted by thoughts, feelings, and sensations. The restless chatter of the mind tends to diminish as one learns to attend to the simple focus of breathing.

Practicing this type of meditation once or twice a day for fifteen or twenty minutes often results in a dynamic new awareness, in which the mind is alert and attentive yet also tranquil. This "meditative mood" tends to carry over into daily experience, affording more clarity and flexibility in daily decisions and actions. Your mind becomes better able to concentrate in the midst of distractions, and you become more capable of relaxing in high-pressure situations. You begin to enjoy the simpler pleasures in life, and your attitude improves dramatically. With daily practice, the meditative frame of mind becomes second nature, replacing automatic, sometimes damaging reactivity, and responses that are not in your best interests. As Dr. Joan Borysenko, former director of Boston's Mind/Body Clinic, writes in *Minding the Body, Mending the Mind,* "The final goal of meditation is to be constantly conscious of experience so that relaxation and peace of mind become the norm rather than the exception." Meditation is a valuable part of cancer treatment programs, and it is being used in many clinics.

Relaxation Training

Relaxation training has similar effects, producing a sense of calm and a heightened, peaceful awareness. The technique involves intentionally relaxing your muscles, starting with the small muscles of the face and then working your way down to your neck, arms, chest, and so on. One technique is to momentarily tighten each muscle group and then let it go to achieve total relaxation. A second method is to imagine that your breathing can actually carry out tension. You simply try to picture your inhalation carrying cool, refreshing air into your face and neck, for example, and then picture all the tension leaving these areas as you breathe out. Then use the same mental image for each muscle group in sequence. Many cancer clinics have classes in relaxation training. In addition to physical relaxation, these offer instruction that helps the patient visualize the process of overcoming the tumor and reaching health. Guided imagery is the same method of harnessing mental energy that is used by star athletes.

Relaxation training has been shown to influence the immune systems of healthy people, and of cancer patients during chemotherapy. Whether this gives real protection against cancer remains to be seen. Clearly it can reduce fear, tension, and anxiety, and increase confidence and optimism. Relaxation training and meditation don't have the drawbacks of double martinis and cigarettes, nor the side effects of prescription drugs that many people use to deal with stress.

Support from Others

People with strong social support have less risk of getting cancer and better survival rates if cancer does occur. Knowing there are others you can turn to gives you a sense of stability and allows you to deal more effectively with life's challenges. Sharing your fears and frustrations is invaluable. Being around healthy and positive people also is important. They can give you perspective, a non-judgmental ear, and a good laugh at a crucial moment.

Though it may be difficult at first to ask for, or even to accept help from others, doing so can be a wonderful part of healing. During one man's treatments, he and his wife developed a care team, through the help of their church and friends. These people helped him get from work to radiation appointments, and to visits to his doctor. A woman returning home from the hospital received a month's worth of vegetarian meals, delivered to her home each evening at 6:00 P.M. Her neighbor had circulated a sign-up sheet among their friends. It was a simple matter for each household to make a few extra servings on their appointed day, and to take over to her enough for supper, and for lunch the next day.

Everyone finds support in his or her own way. Some people get reassurance from a priest, a minister, or a rabbi. Others prefer their family members, cats, dogs, or photographs. For more than twenty years, oncologist Rachel Naomi Remen has used a small stone for cancer patients. It sound odd, but it proves very reassuring. Here is how it works for people who undergo radiation, chemotherapy, or surgery. She suggests that the cancer patient meet with close friends the day before the procedure. Prior to this meeting, the person finds an ordinary stone, of a size to fit in the palm of the hand. Sitting together in a circle, each person, in turn, holds the stone while sharing their experience of a time when they, too, faced a crisis. They express a quality (such as determination or faith) that they wish to accompany the patient to his or her procedure, saying, "I put determination into this stone for you." As the person enters the procedure the next day, he or she is accompanied by the stone, which may be taped to the hand or the foot. The stone is then a symbol of the love and prayers that go with the cancer patient during this experience. Dr. Remen's book or tape *Kitchen Table Wisdom* is a wealth of touching, enlightening, and funny stories that can help with the experience of cancer.

Our most challenging experiences also can be the most rewarding. Through them we are inspired (or pushed) to take important steps we would not otherwise have made. It is tremendously life-affirming to take control of your own body, recognizing the power you do have. When you take charge of the situation through exercise, food choices, meditation, relaxation, and enlisting the support of others, the returns are immense.

10

Putting It All Together

Scientific research continues to bring new insights on the surprising links between nutrition and cancer. In research studies, scientists help people change their diets and then measure how nutrients enter their bloodstreams and power up anticancer defenses. Other researchers examine cancer-fighting immune cells under the microscope and see how various nutrients help or hinder them. Almost daily, we learn more about how to knock out the free radicals that can cause cancer, how to readjust the hormones that can affect cancer risk, and how to strengthen our resistance.

We already know more than enough to get started. At first, the basic principles seem simple—cut the fat, boost the fiber, bring in the antioxidant vitamins, be careful about alcohol. But we have applied these and other principles in a way that is much more effective than you may have imagined. As you'll see in the recipes that follow, we have taken humble foods—vegetables, fruits, whole grains, legumes—and allowed their full healing powers to blossom.

Incorporated into wonderful recipes, they are also delights for your taste buds. And a cancer-fighting menu has other benefits you may not have expected. It will likely give you extra energy, trim your waistline, and lower your cholesterol level—*by a great deal.* If you have high blood pressure or diabetes, the same foods that fight cancer will do wonders for these problems, too.

A dietary approach has one other vitally important advantage. Unlike a radiation beam that affects only the organ it is focused upon, or surgery that benefits only one patient at a time, a diet change helps the whole family. As everyone joins together to enjoy a hearty meal, they are also getting healthier—whether they are aware of it or not. And as healthy foods are placed on the lunch or dinner table, parents give their children—and each other—a wonderful gift that will literally last a lifetime.

Let me encourage you to venture into a menu change with the sense that you really are trying some new things. As you experiment with recipes, or perhaps new menu items at restaurants, you'll find some winners, some exotic tastes, and even an occasional dud. That's what experimenting is all about. When you find the foods you really love, they'll soon become fast friends. And please share your new knowledge with others. They'll profit, just as you have.

We wish you the very best of success in your new endeavor, and the very best of health.

11

Cooking Tips and Techniques

In this chapter you will find recipes, menus, and tips to help you prepare delicious meals for cancer prevention and overall good health. You'll find practical suggestions for menu planning and shopping, and sample menus based on the recipes in this book. "Stocking Your Pantry" provides suggestions for staple ingredients as well as convenient instant meals to keep on hand, and the Glossary lists foods that may be new to you. The recipes included in this section are quick and easy to prepare, with ingredients that are available in most grocery stores. Many of the recipes are for healthful versions of familiar foods, and each of the recipes includes a nutrient analysis.

Planning a Menu

As with many other tasks in life, a little planning helps with meal preparation, too. You will be amazed at the amount of time and money you save when you plan weekly menus and shop for a week at a time. You'll spend less time looking for parking and standing in line, and by planning ahead you'll spend less money on impulse items and instant meals. You'll also be delighted when you begin cooking that all the ingredients you need will be on hand.

Set aside a bit of time and find a quiet spot to plan a one-week menu. Your menu plan does not have to specify every item for every meal. Breakfasts, especially during the week, will probably be much the same from day to day: fruits, whole grain cereals, and breads. For lunches, leftovers make perfect instant meals. Soup (either homemade or commercially prepared) is another quick and nutritious option. Add whole grain bread and salad mix sprinkled with seasoned rice vinegar for a meal in minutes! Bean or grain salads are also excellent lunch foods that can be prepared in quantity and kept on hand for a quick meal. Thus your lunch menu plan should include a couple of soups and two or three salads. For dinners, plan four main dishes, prepared in large enough quantities to provide at least two meals. Add whole grains such as brown rice or bulgur wheat, and vegetables for complete, satisfying meals.

A Sample Menu Plan

This flexible menu plan does not specify exact meals for each day of the week. The indicated meals can be prepared according to your time and taste. At the same time, it provides you with the assurance that the ingredients for any of the meals will be available when you need them. Use this menu plan to make a shopping list.

SAMPLE MENU PLAN

Breakfasts
>   fresh fruit: blueberries, cantaloupes, oranges
>   toast: whole wheat raisin, multigrain
>   hot cereal: oatmeal, ten-grain cereal, cracked wheat
>   cold cereal: shredded wheat, muesli

Lunches
>   soups: Green Velvet Soup, Lentil Soup, Gazpacho
>   salads: Tex-Mex Salad, Fresh Broccoli Salad, Red Potato Salad

Dinners
>   Black Bean Chili
>   Polenta
>   Carrot, Beet, and Jicama Salad

Dinners (continued)

Thai Vegetables
Brown Rice
Ginger Noodles

Creamy Beet Soup
Kasha with Broccoli and Black Bean Sauce
Mixed Greens with Apples and Walnuts

Eggplant Manicotti
Minestrone
Fresh Broccoli Salad

Making a Shopping List

Use your menu plan to prepare a shopping list. Look up the recipes you have chosen and note the ingredients that you'll need to purchase. Add a variety of fresh vegetables and fruits, whole grains, and breads to round out your meals. Check the refrigerator, freezer, and pantry to see what staples need to be restocked (see "Stocking Your Pantry" on page 138). These might include condiments, spices, baking supplies, canned foods, frozen foods, and beverages.

To streamline your shopping trip, arrange the foods on your list in categories that reflect the departments in your grocery store, such as fresh produce, grains, dried beans, canned fruits and vegetables, and frozen foods.

SAMPLE SHOPPING LIST

Fresh Produce

oranges	prewashed spinach	green beans
bananas	carrots	green bell peppers
cantaloupes	celery	red bell peppers
blueberries	portobello	tomatoes
other seasonal fruits	mushrooms	fresh beets
prewashed salad	sweet potatoes	red potatoes
mix	green onions	broccoli

collard greens   yellow onions   jicamas
zucchini   red onions   other seasonal
avocados   garlic   vegetables

Breakfast Cereals

oatmeal   multigrain cereal   shredded wheat

Grains and Pasta

rolled oats   polenta   elbow macaroni
couscous   whole wheat pastry
brown basmati rice   flour

Dried Beans and Peas

lentils   pinto beans   split peas

Canned Vegetables and Fruits

15-ounce can   15-ounce can   roasted red
  diced beets   kidney beans   peppers
28-ounce can   15-ounce can   tomato juice
  crushed tomatoes   garbanzo beans

Packaged Foods

ramen soups   fortified soy milk
                    or rice milk

Refrigerated Foods

tofu   flour tortillas

Bread

whole wheat bread

Salad Dressing, Vinegar, and Condiments

reduced-sodium   balsamic vinegar
  soy sauce

Herbs and Spices

chili powder   oregano

Frozen Foods

orange juice   apple juice   chopped spinach
  concentrate   concentrate

Seasonal Eating

Seasonal eating refers to choosing fruits and vegetables when they are fresh and in season. By doing so, you will enjoy better-tasting, more nutritious produce and cut your food costs at the same time. Seasonal produce tastes better because it is usually picked at its prime. It hasn't spent weeks in transit from the other side of the equator, or months in cold storage, where it loses moisture, flavor, and nutrients. Ironically, transportation and cold storage, which detract from the flavor and nutritional value of produce, add significantly to its cost.

There are a number of ways to know what foods are in season. Seasonal foods are usually featured in advertisements and in the produce department at your market. Check your store's advertising flyer and look for large end-aisle displays in the produce department. In general you will find that seasonal foods are more reasonably priced than out-of-season produce because of lower storage, shipping, and handling costs. You will also find that when foods are in season, there are often several varieties to choose from. For example, when apples get ripe in autumn, most stores feature several varieties. By spring and summer, however, only the few varieties that can be held in cold storage are available.

Farmers' markets offer an enjoyable way to find out what is in season. The produce at farmers' markets is not only seasonal, but is often organically grown as well. An easy way to obtain seasonal produce is to join a CSA (community-supported agriculture), in which you pay a fee to a local grower who then supplies you with a variety of fresh produce throughout the season. At www.umass.edu/umext/csa/us/StateList.html you can get more information about CSAs, including local listings.

The most basic way of knowing what is in season is to consider what part of the plant a food comes from. During the colder months, foods that are in season generally come from the roots, stems, and leaves of plants. As the weather warms, pods, flowers, and eventually fruits come into season. Fruit, by the way, refers to the seed-bearing portion of a plant, and includes such foods as tomatoes, peppers, avocados, squashes, corn, and eggplant.

Stocking Up

With your shopping list in hand, you will be ready to stock up quickly and conveniently for the whole week. Make sure you have eaten *before* you head for the store. Shopping on an empty stomach can override the best of intentions and lead to impulsive purchases of less-than-nutritious foods.

Most processed foods have nutrition labels and ingredient lists that provide you with useful information for making healthful food choices. The nutrition label indicates the size of a single serving and the number of calories as well as the amount of fat, protein, sugar, fiber, and salt in that serving. You can also gather a lot of useful information by reading through the ingredients list. The ingredients are listed in order of prominence in the food: the ingredient present in the greatest amount is first on the list, and so forth. Thus, if fat or sugar appears near the top of the list, you know that these are major ingredients. The ingredients list also indicates the presence of artificial flavors, artificial colors, preservatives, and other additives you may wish to avoid.

As you read through the ingredients list, be aware of the many different forms of sugar that may be in food. Sucrose, fructose, dextrose, corn syrup, honey, and malt are just a few, and in general, any ingredients that end with "ose" are sugars. If a product contains several different types of sugar it is likely that sugar is a major ingredient, even if it isn't the first item on the list.

You should also avoid foods that contain hydrogenated oils. These oils have been processed to make them solid, or saturated, and like other saturated fats, they can raise blood cholesterol levels and increase the risk of heart disease.

In addition to nutrition labels and ingredients lists, foods may contain other nutrition claims, such as "fat-free," "low cholesterol," or "lite." The definitions of these terms, as outlined by the U.S. Food and Drug Administration, are given in the following list.

Light (lite). May refer to calories, fat, or sodium. Contains a third fewer calories, or no more than half the fat of the higher-calorie, higher-fat version; or no more than half the sodium of the higher-sodium version.

Calorie-free. Contains fewer than 5 calories per serving.

Fat-free. Contains fewer than 0.5 gram of fat per serving.

Low-fat. Contains 3 grams of fat (or less) per serving.

Reduced or less fat. At least 25 percent less fat per serving than the higher-fat version.

Cholesterol-free. Contains fewer than 2 milligrams of cholesterol and 2 grams (or less) of saturated fat per serving.

Low cholesterol. Contains 20 milligrams of cholesterol (or less) and 2 grams of saturated fat (or less) per serving.

Reduced cholesterol. At least 25 percent less cholesterol than the higher-cholesterol version and 2 grams (or less) or saturated fat per serving.

Sodium-free. Contains fewer than 5 milligrams of sodium per serving and no sodium chloride in ingredients.

Very low sodium. Contains 35 milligrams of sodium (or less) per serving.

Low sodium. Contains 140 milligrams of sodium (or less) per serving.

Stocking Your Pantry

BASIC INGREDIENTS AND QUICK FOODS

Produce

yellow onions	carrots, baby	broccoli
red onions	carrots	kale or collard
garlic	celery	greens
red potatoes	prewashed salad	apples
russet potatoes	mix	oranges
green cabbage	prewashed spinach	bananas

Grains and Grain Products

short grain brown rice	whole wheat flour	rice flour
long grain brown rice	whole wheat pastry flour	barley flour
bulgur	unbleached flour	whole wheat cous- cous
	potato flour	rolled oats

polenta
cornmeal
eggless pasta

cold breakfast cere-
als without added
fat or sugars

hot breakfast
cereals

Dried Beans, Lentils, and Peas

pinto beans
black beans
lentils
split peas

black bean flakes:
Fantastic Foods,
Taste Adventure

pinto bean flakes:
Fantastic Foods,
Taste Adventure

Canned Foods

basic beans (pinto,
garbanzo, kidney,
black)
prepared beans
(vegetarian chili,
baked beans,
refried beans)

tomato products
(crushed toma-
toes, tomato
sauce, tomato
paste)
vegetables (corn,
beets, water-
packed roasted
red peppers)

vegetarian soups
vegetarian pasta
sauce (preferably
fat-free)
salsa

Frozen Foods

unsweetened juice
concentrates
(apple, orange,
white grape)
frozen bananas

frozen berries
frozen vegetables
(corn, peas, Ital-
ian green beans,
broccoli)

chopped onions
frozen diced bell
peppers

Nuts, Seeds, and Dried Fruit

peanut butter

tahini (sesame
butter)

raisins

Breads, Crackers, and Snack Foods

whole grain bread
(may be frozen)
whole wheat pita
bread

corn tortillas
(may be frozen)
whole wheat
tortillas (may be
frozen)

fat-free snack
foods (crackers,
rice cakes, pop-
corn cakes, baked
tortilla chips,
pretzels)

Convenience Foods

vegetarian soup cups	silken tofu	baked tofu
vegetarian ramen soups	vegetarian burgers, cold cuts, hot dogs	textured vegetable protein

Condiments and Seasonings

herbs and spices	molasses	fat-free salad dressing
reduced-sodium soy sauce	maple syrup	eggless mayonnaise (Vegenaise, Nayonaise)
cider vinegar	raw or turbinado sugar	
balsamic vinegar	baking soda	
seasoned rice vinegar	low-sodium baking powder (Feather-weight)	stone-ground mustard
vegetable broth		catsup
vegetable oil spray	spreadable fruit	

Beverages

fortified soy milk/rice milk	plain or calcium enriched juices	hot beverages (herbal teas, Cafix, Postum, Pero)

Meal Preparation

With your menu and ingredients on hand, you will be able to prepare satisfying meals quickly and conveniently. You may wish to prepare several different menu items in a single cooking session as a further time-saver.

You will notice that most of the recipes in this book provide six to eight servings. As a result, you will probably have food left over that can be used to provide one or more extra meals. In this way, the menu you create may actually provide meals for more than a week, with no additional shopping, planning, or cooking!

Another time-saver is to make slight modifications to the food you've already prepared so it has a different appearance the second or third time you serve it. In this way you can have maximum variety with minimum preparation. The Black Bean Dip (see page 172) is a good example. Start out by preparing a double batch and serve it as a dip or as a burrito filling as indicated in the recipe. For a second meal, add a bit more water, and serve it as a sauce for steamed red potatoes or broccoli. Or add even more water, or vegetable broth and a few chopped green onions, to turn it into a delicious soup.

Foods that take a bit of time to cook can be prepared in large enough quantities to provide for several meals. Brown rice is a good example. Once cooked, it can be easily reheated in a microwave or on the stovetop and served as a side dish with a variety of recipes. It also can be added to soups and stews, or used as a filling in a burrito or a wrap.

Cooking Techniques

Vegetables

The secret to preparing vegetables is to cook them only as much as is needed to tenderize them and bring out their best flavor. The following methods are quick and easy and enhance the flavor and texture of vegetables.

Steaming. A collapsible steamer rack can turn any pot into a vegetable steamer. Heat about 1 inch of water in a pot. Arrange the prepared vegetables in a single layer on a steamer rack and place them in the pot over the boiling water. Cover the pot with a lid and cook until just tender.

Braising. This technique is identical to sautéing, except that a fat-free liquid is used in place of oil. It is particularly useful for mellowing the flavor of vegetables such as onions and garlic. Heat approximately ½ cup of water, vegetable broth, or wine (the liquid you use will depend on the recipe) in a large pan or skillet. Add the vegetables and cook over high heat, stirring occasionally, adding small amounts of additional liquid if needed, until the vegetables are tender. This will take about five minutes for onions.

Grilling. High heat seals in the flavors of vegetables and adds its own distinctive flavor as well. Vegetables can be grilled on a barbecue or electric grill, or on the stove using a nonstick grill pan. Cut all the foods that will be grilled together into a uniform size. Preheat the grill, then add the vegetables. Cook over medium-high heat, turning occasionally with a spatula until uniformly browned and tender.

Roasting. A simple and delicious way to prepare vegetables is to roast them in a very hot oven (450°F). Toss the vegetables with seasonings and a small amount of olive oil if desired. Spread them in a single layer on a baking sheet and place them in the preheated oven until tender.

Microwave. A microwave oven provides an easy method for cooking vegetables, particularly those that take a long time to cook with other methods. Another benefit of microwave cooking for vegetables is that they cook quickly with little or no water, minimizing loss of nutrients. Try the recipes for yams, potatoes, and winter squash on page 198.

Grains

Whole grains are a mainstay of a healthful diet. The term "whole grain" refers to grains that have been minimally processed, leaving the bran and germ intact. As a result, whole grains provide significantly more nutrients, including protein, vitamins, and minerals, than refined grains. In addition, whole grains are an excellent source of fiber. Some fairly common whole grains include whole wheat berries, cracked wheat and bulgur, whole wheat flour, brown rice, rolled oats, whole barley, and barley flour. Some of the less common grains that are slowly making their way into the mainstream are quinoa, amaranth, kamut, and teff.

Grains should be stored in a cool, dry location. If the outer bran layer has been disturbed by crushing or grinding, as in making flour or rolled oats, the grain should be used within two to three months. Grains with the outer bran layer intact remain viable and nutritious for several years if properly stored.

When cooking grains, the following tips are useful:

- The easiest way to cook most grains is to simmer them, loosely covered, on the stovetop.
- Lightly roasting grains in a dry skillet before cooking enhances their nutty flavor and gives them a lighter texture. The flavor of millet is particularly enhanced by roasting.
- Grains should not be stirred during cooking, unless the recipe indicates otherwise. They will be lighter and fluffier if left alone.
- When cooking grains, make enough for several meals.

Cooked grains can be reheated in a microwave or on the stovetop.

- An easy way to reheat grains on the stove is to place them in a vegetable steamer over boiling water.
- Fine-textured grains such as couscous and bulgur are fluffier when they are not cooked. Simply pour boiling water over the grain, then cover and let stand for fifteen to twenty minutes. Fluff the grain with a fork before serving.

Legumes

The term "legume" refers to dried beans and peas such as soybeans, black beans, pinto beans, garbanzos or chickpeas, lentils, and split peas. Legumes may be purchased dried, canned, and in some cases, frozen or dehydrated. Dried beans are inexpensive and easy to cook. If you don't have the time to cook dried beans, canned beans are a good alternative. Kidney beans, garbanzo beans, pinto beans, black beans, and many others are available, including some in low-sodium varieties. For an even quicker meal, vegetarian baked beans, chili beans, and refried beans are available in the canned food section of most supermarkets.

Recently a few companies have introduced precooked, dehydrated beans. These cook in about five minutes. Pinto beans, black beans, split peas, and lentils are some of the varieties available. Check your local natural food store for these.

Note the following tips for cooking dried beans:

- Sort through the beans, discard any debris, then rinse thoroughly.
- Soaking beans before cooking reduces their cooking time and increases their digestibility. Soak at least four hours, then pour off soak water and add fresh water for cooking.
- Cook in a large pot with plenty of water. Cover the pot loosely. Use medium-low heat to maintain a low simmer. Check occasionally, adding more water if needed.
- A Crock-Pot is an ideal place to cook beans. The slow, even heat ensures thorough cooking. Start with boiling water and use the highest setting for quickest cooking. For slower cooking, start with cold water and use the highest setting.

COOKING DRIED BEANS AND PEAS

BEANS (1 CUP DRY)	AMOUNT OF WATER	COOKING TIME	YIELD
Adzuki beans	3 cups	1½ hours	2¼ cups
Black beans	3 cups	1½ hours	2¼ cups
Black-eyed peas	3 cups	1 hour	2 cups
Chickpeas (garbanzos)	4 cups	2–3 hours	2½ cups
Great Northern beans	3½ cups	2 hours	2 cups
Kidney beans	3 cups	2 hours	2 cups
Lentils	3 cups	1 hour	2¼ cups
Lima beans	2 cups	1½ hours	1½ cups
Navy beans	3 cups	2 hours	2 cups
Pinto beans	3 cups	2½ hours	2¼ cups
Red beans	3 cups	3 hours	2 cups
Soybeans	4 cups	3 hours	2½ cups
Split peas	3 cups	1 hour	2½ cups

- Beans can be cooked very quickly in a pressure cooker. Follow the instructions that came with the cooker.
- Beans should be thoroughly cooked. They should smash easily when pressed between thumb and forefinger.
- Salt toughens the skins of beans and increases the cooking time. It should not be added until the beans are tender.
- Cooked beans may be frozen in airtight containers for later use.

Cutting Fat

Foods that are high in fat are also high in calories. In addition to causing unwanted weight gain, a high-fat diet increases your risk for heart disease, adult-onset diabetes, and several forms of cancer. By switching to a plant-based diet you will reduce your intake of fat considerably. The following tips will help you reduce your fat intake even further.

- Choose cooking techniques that do not employ added fat. Baking, grilling, and oven roasting are great alternatives to frying.
- Another fat-cutting cooking trick is to sauté in a liquid such as water or vegetable broth whenever possible. Heat about ½ cup of water in a skillet (preferably nonstick) and add the vegetables to be sautéed. Cook over high heat, stirring frequently, until the vegetables are tender. This will take about five minutes. Add a bit more water if necessary to prevent sticking.
- Add onions and garlic to soups and stews at the beginning of the cooking time so their flavors will mellow without sautéing.
- When oil is absolutely necessary to prevent sticking, lightly apply a vegetable oil spray. Another alternative is to start with a very small amount of oil (1 to 2 teaspoons), then add water or vegetable broth as needed to keep the food from sticking.
- Nonstick pots and pans allow foods to be prepared with little or no fat.
- Choose fat-free dressings for salads. In addition to commercially prepared dressings, seasoned rice vinegar makes a tasty fat-free dressing straight out of the bottle.
- Avoid deep-fried foods and fat-laden pastries. Check your market for low-fat and no-fat alternatives.
- Replace the oil in salad dressing recipes with seasoned rice vinegar, vegetable broth, bean cooking liquid, or water. For a thicker dressing, whisk in a small amount of potato flour.
- Sesame Seasoning (see page 175) is low in fat and delicious on grains, potatoes, and steamed vegetables. Fat-free salad dressing also may be used as a topping for cooked vegetables.
- Applesauce, mashed banana, prune puree, or canned pumpkin may be substituted for all or part of the fat in many baked goods.

Quick Meal and Snack Ideas

- Fresh soybeans (edamame) make a delicious snack or meal addition. Find them in the frozen-vegetable section of the supermarket, and prepare according to package directions.
- For an instant green salad use prewashed salad mix and commercially prepared fat-free dressing. Add some canned kidney beans or garbanzo beans for a more substantial meal.

- Baby carrots make a convenient, healthful snack. Try them plain or with a prepared hummus dip or Black Bean Dip (see page 172).
- Ramen soup is quick and satisfying. Add some chopped, fresh vegetables for a heartier soup.
- Keep a selection of vegetarian soup cups on hand. These are great for quick meals, especially when you're traveling.
- Burritos are quick to make and very portable. They can be eaten hot or cold. For a simple burrito, spread fat-free refried beans on a flour tortilla, add prewashed salad mix and salsa, and roll it up.
- Mix fat-free refried beans with an equal amount of salsa for a delicious bean dip. Serve with baked tortilla chips or fresh vegetables.
- Baked Tofu Sandwiches (see page 161) are quick and easy to make. Serve them with Fresh Tomatoes with Basil (see page 168).
- A wide variety of fat-free vegetarian cold cuts are available in many supermarkets and natural-foods stores. These make quick and easy sandwiches.
- Rice cakes and popcorn cakes make great snack foods. Spread them with apple butter or spreadable fruit.
- Drain garbanzo beans and spoon onto a piece of pita bread. Top with prewashed salad mix and fat-free salad dressing for a quick pocket sandwich.
- Heat a fat-free vegetarian burger patty in the toaster oven. Serve it on a whole grain bun with mustard, ketchup or barbecue sauce, and lettuce. Add sliced red onion and tomato if desired.
- Keep baked or steamed potatoes in the refrigerator. For a quick meal, heat a potato in the microwave and top it with Black Bean Chili (see page 186).
- Arrange chunks of fresh fruit on skewers for quick fruit kabobs.
- Frozen grapes make a refreshing summer snack. To prepare, remove them from the stems and freeze, loosely packed, in an airtight container.
- Frozen bananas make cool snacks or creamy desserts. Peel the bananas, break into chunks, and freeze in airtight containers.

12

Menus for a Week

DAY 1

Breakfast

    cold cereal or hot Multigrain Cereal (page 155)

    fortified soy milk or rice milk

    fresh fruit

    herb tea

Lunch

    Zucchini Pockets (page 163)

    Tex-Mex Salad (page 169)

    fresh fruit

Dinner

    Black Bean Chili (page 186)

    Brown Rice (page 157)

    Fresh Broccoli Salad (page 168)

    Fresh Peach Crisp (page 209)

DAY 2

Breakfast

French Toast (page 153)

Corn Butter (page 172)

maple syrup or spreadable fruit

fresh fruit

herb tea

Lunch

Lentil Soup (page 185)

Fresh Tomatoes with Basil (page 168)

whole grain bread

Dinner

Eggplant Manicotti (page 194)

Minestrone (page 182)

Garlic Bread (page 207)

Blueberry Pudding (page 212)

DAY 3

Breakfast

Blueberry Buckwheat Pancakes (page 151)

Corn Butter (page 172)

maple syrup or spreadable fruit

fresh fruit

herb tea

Lunch

Lima Bean Soup (page 183)

whole grain bread or roll

Spinach Salad with Orange Sesame Dressing (page 171)

Dinner

Cabbage Rolls (page 187)

Mixed Greens with Apples and Walnuts (page 170)

Brown Rice (page 157)

Holiday Fruitcake (page 212)

DAY 4

Breakfast
> Oatmeal Waffles (page 152)
> fresh fruit or spreadable fruit
> herb tea

Lunch
> Green Velvet Soup (page 180)
> Garlic Bread (page 207)
> Tex-Mex Salad (page 169)

Dinner
> Black Bean Pueblo Pie (using leftover Black Bean Chili) (page 193)
> Carrot, Beet, and Jicama Salad (page 171)
> Blueberry Freeze (page 213)

DAY 5

Breakfast
> cold cereal or hot Multigrain Cereal (page 155)
> fortified soy milk or rice milk
> fresh fruit
> herb tea

Lunch
> Gazpacho (page 185)
> Broccoli Burritos (page 166)
> watermelon

Dinner
> Collard Greens with Portobello Mushrooms (page 190)
> basmati rice
> Fruit Gel (page 211)

DAY 6

Breakfast

    Zucchini Scramble (page 153)

    whole grain toast with Corn Butter (page 172)

    Blueberry Sauce (page 179) or spreadable fruit

    herb tea

Lunch

    Red Beans and Rice (page 191)

    Mixed Greens with Apples and Walnuts (page 170)

    fresh fruit

Dinner

    Lasagna (page 192)

    French Bread with Roasted Garlic (page 206)

    green salad with fat-free dressing

    Prune Whip (page 210)

DAY 7

Breakfast

    Blueberry Muesli (page 156) or Sweet Potato Pudding (page 156)

    fortified soy milk or rice milk

    fresh fruit

    herb tea

Lunch

    Bean Burger (page 163)

    baby carrots with Creamy Dill Dressing (page 177)

Dinner

    Thai Vegetables (page 188)

    Ginger Noodles (page 160)

    Carrots in Orange Sauce (page 200)

    Berry Cobbler (page 209)

13

The Recipes

BREAKFASTS

Blueberry Buckwheat Pancakes
MAKES 16 3-INCH PANCAKES

In this recipe, buckwheat and blueberries team up to make a terrific tasting, health-protecting breakfast.

½ cup buckwheat flour
½ cup cornmeal
½ teaspoon baking powder
¼ teaspoon baking soda
¼ teaspoon salt
1 ripe banana, mashed

2 tablespoons maple syrup
1 tablespoon cider vinegar
1 cup fortified soy milk or rice milk
1 cup fresh or frozen blueberries
vegetable oil cooking spray

Combine buckwheat flour, cornmeal, baking powder, baking soda, and salt.

In a large bowl, combine mashed banana, maple syrup, vinegar, and milk. Add flour mixture, stirring just enough to remove any lumps and make a pourable batter. Stir in blueberries and add a bit more milk if the batter seems too thick.

Preheat a nonstick skillet or griddle, and then spray lightly with vegetable oil cooking spray. Pour batter (about ¼ cup per pancake) onto the heated surface and cook until tops bubble. Turn pancakes carefully with a spatula and cook until the second sides are browned, about 1 minute. Serve immediately.

Per pancake: 52 calories; 1 g protein; 11 g carbohydrate; 0.45 g fat;
1 g fiber; 56 mg sodium; calories from protein: 9%;
calories from carbohydrates: 83%; calories from fats: 8%

● ● ●

Whole Wheat Barley Cakes
MAKES ABOUT 16 3-INCH PANCAKES

½ cup barley flour
½ cup whole wheat pastry flour
½ teaspoon baking soda
¼ teaspoon salt
1¼ cups fortified soy milk or rice
   milk

1 tablespoon maple syrup
1 tablespoon cider vinegar
1½ teaspoons canola oil
vegetable oil cooking spray

Stir barley flour, pastry flour, baking soda, and salt together in one bowl. In a separate bowl mix milk, maple syrup, vinegar, and oil. Combine the two mixtures and stir just enough to obtain a smooth batter.

Heat a nonstick skillet, then lightly spray it with vegetable oil spray. Pour batter (about ¼ cup per pancake) onto the heated surface and cook until the edges are dry and the tops bubble. Turn carefully with a spatula and cook until the second sides are golden brown, about 1 minute.

Per pancake: 57 calories; 2 g protein; 10 g carbohydrate; 1 g fat; 2 g fiber;
110 mg sodium; calories from protein: 14%;
calories from carbohydrates: 70%; calories from fats: 16%

● ● ●

Oatmeal Waffles
MAKES 6 WAFFLES

These easily prepared waffles are a delicious way to add healthful oats to your diet.

2 cups rolled oats
2 cups water
1 banana
¼ teaspoon salt
1 tablespoon maple syrup

1 teaspoon vanilla
fresh fruit, spreadable fruit, or
   maple syrup for serving
vegetable oil cooking spray

Preheat waffle iron to medium-high.

Combine oats, water, banana, salt, maple syrup, and vanilla in a blender. Blend on high speed until completely smooth.

Lightly spray waffle iron with cooking spray. Pour in enough batter to just barely reach edges and cook until golden brown, 5 to 10 minutes. without lifting lid.

Note: The batter should be pourable. If it becomes too thick as it stands, add a bit more water to achieve desired consistency.

Serve with fresh fruit, spreadable fruit, or syrup.

Per waffle: 130 calories; 5 g protein; 25 g carbohydrate; 2 g fat; 3 g fiber;
90 mg sodium; calories from protein: 14%;
calories from carbohydrates: 74%; calories from fats: 12%

• • •

French Toast
MAKES 6 SLICES

This cholesterol-free French toast tastes great as it adds beneficial soy and whole wheat to your diet.

1 cup fortified soy milk (plain or vanilla)	1 teaspoon vanilla
	½ teaspoon cinnamon
¼ cup whole wheat pastry flour	6 slices whole grain bread
1 tablespoon maple syrup	vegetable oil cooking spray

Combine milk, flour, maple syrup, vanilla, and cinnamon in a blender. Blend until smooth, then pour into a flat dish.

Soak bread slices in batter until soft but not soggy. The amount of time this takes will vary depending on the bread used.

Cook in an oil-sprayed nonstick skillet over medium heat until first side is golden brown, about 3 minutes. Turn carefully with a spatula and cook second side until brown, about 3 minutes.

Per slice: 129 calories; 6 g protein; 23 g carbohydrate; 2 g fat; 4 g fiber;
191 mg sodium; calories from protein: 17%;
calories from carbohydrates: 68%; calories from fats: 15%

• • •

Zucchini Scramble
MAKES 4 1-CUP SERVINGS

This quick scramble makes a delicious breakfast. Serve it with English muffins, warm tortillas, or toasted French bread.

$\frac{1}{2}$ cup water
1 onion, chopped
2 garlic cloves, minced
2 medium zucchini, finely diced
   (about 2 cups)

$\frac{1}{2}$ pound firm tofu, diced
1 teaspoon chili powder
1 to 2 tablespoons reduced-sodium
   soy sauce
about $\frac{1}{2}$ cup salsa (optional)

Heat the water in a large nonstick skillet. Add onion and garlic. Cook over high heat, stirring often, until soft, about 5 minutes.

Add zucchini, tofu, and chili powder. Reduce heat and cook, stirring often, until zucchini is tender, about 5 minutes. Add a small amount of additional water if necessary to prevent sticking.

Stir in soy sauce. Top with salsa if desired.

Per 1-cup serving: 98 calories; 8 g protein; 13 g carbohydrate; 3 g fat; 4 g fiber; 316 mg sodium; calories from protein: 29%; calories from carbohydrates: 46%; calories from fats: 25%

• • •

Braised Potatoes
MAKES 4 1-CUP SERVINGS

Serve these potatoes with Black Bean Chili (page 186) and spicy salsa for a real eye-opener breakfast. For a more traditional breakfast, try them with Zucchini Scramble (page 153).

4 large red or Yukon Gold potatoes
$\frac{1}{2}$ cup water
4 teaspoons reduced-sodium soy
   sauce

1 onion, chopped
1 teaspoon chili powder
$\frac{1}{8}$ teaspoon freshly ground black
   pepper

Scrub potatoes, but do not peel. Cut into $\frac{1}{4}$-inch-thick slices and steam over boiling water until just tender when pierced with a sharp knife, about 10 minutes.

Heat $\frac{1}{2}$ cup water and 2 teaspoons of the soy sauce in a large nonstick skillet. Add onion and cook until soft, about 5 minutes.

Add cooked potatoes, chili powder, and remaining soy sauce. Stir gently to mix, then cook over medium heat for 5 minutes, stirring occasionally. Sprinkle with black pepper.

Per 1-cup serving: 159 calories; 4 g protein; 37 g carbohydrate; 0.18 g fat; 4 g fiber; 240 mg sodium; calories from protein: 9%; calories from carbohydrates: 90%; calories from fats: 1%

• • •

Apple Cinnamon Oatmeal

MAKES 2 1-CUP SERVINGS

1   cup rolled oats, regular or quick-   1⅓ cups water
    cooking   ½ teaspoon cinnamon
⅔ cup apple juice concentrate   ½ cup raisins or currants (optional)

Combine oats, apple juice concentrate, water, and cinnamon in a sauce-pan. Bring to a simmer, then cover and cook 3 minutes. Remove from heat and stir in raisins, if using. Set stand 3 minutes before serving.

Per ½-cup serving: 296 calories; 7 g protein; 62 g carbohydrate; 2 g fat;
4 g fiber; 22 mg sodium; calories from protein: 9%;
calories from carbohydrates: 82%; calories from fats: 9%

• • •

Multigrain Cereal

MAKES 2½ 1-CUP SERVINGS

Multigrain hot cereals provide great flavor as well as the nutritional benefits of several whole grains. A variety of multigrain cereal mixes are available in natural food stores and many supermarkets. One of the most delicious and most widely distributed is Bob's Red Mill 10 Grain Cereal (see Glossary). Use this method for cooking any of these hearty, satisfying breakfast cereals.

1   cup multigrain cereal mix   3 cups boiling water
½ teaspoon salt (optional)

Stir cereal and salt into boiling water in a saucepan. Cover loosely and simmer, stirring occasionally, for 7 minutes.

Remove from heat and let stand, covered, for 10 minutes before serving.

Health hint: By gradually reducing the amount of salt you add, you can re-educate your taste buds so that the cereal will taste fine with no salt at all.

Per 1-cup serving: 200 calories; 6 g protein; 40 g carbohydrate;
2 g fat; 4 g fiber; 10 to 580 mg sodium (depending on amount
of salt used in recipe); calories from protein: 13%;
calories from carbohydrates: 77%; calories from fats: 10%

• • •

Blueberry Muesli

MAKES ABOUT 3 1-CUP SERVINGS

Muesli is a Swiss breakfast cereal that is a mixture of grains, nuts, and dried fruits. Traditionally, it is soaked overnight in fruit juice, then served with fresh fruit. It may also be served with hot or cold fortified soy milk or rice milk.

2 cups rolled oats	½ cup raisins
¼ cup chopped almonds	2 cups fresh or frozen blueberries
½ cup chopped dried fruit (apples, figs, apricots, etc.)	

Combine oats, almonds, dried fruit, and raisins. Leave whole or grind in a food processor for a finer cereal. Store in an airtight container in the refrigerator.

To serve, mix with fortified soy milk or rice milk, fruit juice, or applesauce. Stir in fresh or frozen blueberries and let stand several minutes before serving.

Per 1-cup muesli with ⅔-cup berries: 458 calories;
13 g protein; 86 g carbohydrate; 10 g fat; 11 g fiber;
16 mg sodium; calories from protein: 12%;
calories from carbohydrates: 70%; calories from fats: 18%

• • •

Sweet Potato Pudding

MAKES ABOUT 3 ½-CUP SERVINGS

Having Sweet Potato Pudding for breakfast is a great way to load up on cancer-fighting beta-carotene. It takes just minutes to make if you keep cooked sweet potatoes or yams on hand (see page 204).

⅓ cup rolled oats	1 cup cooked sweet potato or yam
½ cup fortified soy milk or rice milk	1 tablespoon maple syrup
	¼ teaspoon cinnamon

Combine all ingredients in a blender and blend until smooth.

Per ½-cup serving: 104 calories; 3 g protein; 20 g carbohydrate;
1 g fat; 3 g fiber; 21 mg sodium; calories from protein: 12%;
calories from carbohydrates: 76%; calories from fats: 12%

GRAINS AND PASTAS

Brown Rice

MAKES 3 CUPS OF COOKED RICE (3 1-CUP SERVINGS)

Flavorful and satisfying, brown rice is an excellent source of protective soluble fiber. In the cooking method described below, the rice is toasted, then simmered in plenty of water (like pasta) to enhance its flavor and reduce cooking time.

1 cup short- or long-grain brown rice	4 cups boiling water ½ teaspoon salt

Rinse rice in cool water. Drain off as much water as possible.

Place rice in a saucepan over medium heat, stirring constantly until completely dry, 3 to 5 minutes.

Add boiling water and salt, then cover and simmer until rice is just tender, about 35 minutes. Pour off excess liquid (this can be saved and used as a broth for soups and stews if desired).

Per 1-cup serving: 228 calories; 5 g protein; 48 g carbohydrate;
2 g fat; 2 g fiber; 360 mg sodium; calories from protein: 9%;
calories from carbohydrates: 84%; calories from fats: 7%

• • •

Brown Rice and Barley

MAKES ABOUT 6 1-CUP SERVINGS

The addition of whole barley adds great texture to brown rice. Hulled barley, which is a bit less refined and slightly more nutritious than pearled barley, is sold in many natural food stores.

1 cup short-grain brown rice	1 teaspoon salt
1 cup hulled or pearled barley	

Bring 4 cups water to a boil; add rice, barley, and salt. Reduce heat to a simmer, then cover and cook until grains are tender and all the water is absorbed, about 45 minutes.

Per 1-cup serving: 222 calories; 6 g protein; 46 g carbohydrate;
2 g fat; 6 g fiber; 362 mg sodium; calories from protein: 11%;
calories from carbohydrates: 81%; calories from fats: 8%

• • •

Seasoned Rice

MAKES 2 1-CUP SERVINGS

Serve this tasty rice with steamed or grilled vegetables, or add it to soups for extra texture and flavor.

2 cups hot cooked Brown Rice (page 157)	2 tablespoons Sesame Seasoning (page 175)

Combine cooked rice and Sesame Seasoning and toss gently to mix.

Per 1-cup serving: 274 calories; 8 g protein; 48 g carbohydrate; 6 g fat;
5 g fiber; 146 mg sodium; calories from protein: 11%;
calories from carbohydrates: 69%; calories from fats: 20%

• • •

Bulgur

MAKES 2 1-CUP SERVINGS

Bulgur is made from whole wheat kernels that have been cracked and toasted, giving it a delicious, nutty flavor. It cooks quickly and may be served plain, or in a pilaf or salad. It is sold in natural food stores, and in some supermarkets, usually in the bulk food section.

1 cup uncooked bulgur ½ teaspoon salt	2 cups boiling water

Mix bulgur and salt in a large bowl. Stir in boiling water. Cover and let stand until tender, about 25 minutes.

Alternate cooking method: Stir bulgur and salt into boiling water in a saucepan.

Reduce heat to a simmer, then cover and cook without stirring until bulgur is tender, about 15 minutes.

Per 1-cup serving: 192 calories; 6 g protein; 42 g carbohydrate;
0.8 g fat; 10 g fiber; 436 mg sodium; calories from protein: 13%;
calories from carbohydrates: 84%; calories from fats: 3%

• • •

Whole Wheat Couscous

MAKES 3 1-CUP SERVINGS

Couscous is actually pasta that takes only minutes to prepare. It makes a delicious side dish or salad base. Whole wheat couscous, which contains fiber and more vitamins and minerals than refined couscous, is sold in natural food stores and some supermarkets.

1 cup whole wheat couscous   1½ cups boiling water
½ teaspoon salt

Stir couscous and salt into boiling water in a saucepan. Remove from heat and cover. Let stand 10 to 15 minutes, then fluff with a fork and serve.

> Per 1-cup serving: 200 calories; 6 g protein; 42 g carbohydrate;
> 0.2 g fat; 4 g fiber; 364 mg sodium; calories from protein: 14%;
> calories from carbohydrates: 85%; calories from fats: 1%

• • •

Polenta
MAKES 4 1-CUP SERVINGS

Polenta, or coarsely ground cornmeal, is easy to prepare and tremendously versatile. When it is first cooked it is soft, like Cream of Wheat, and perfect for breakfast topped with fruit and fortified soy milk, or for dinner topped with vegetables and a savory sauce. When chilled, it becomes firm and sliceable, perfect for grilling or sautéing.

5 cups water   1 teaspoon thyme (optional)
1 cup polenta   1 teaspoon oregano (optional)
1 teaspoon salt

Measure water into a large pot, then whisk in polenta, salt, and herbs, if using.

Simmer over medium heat, stirring often, until very thick, about 25 minutes.

Serve hot or transfer to a 9-by-13-inch baking dish and chill until firm.

For grilled polenta, turn cold polenta out of the pan onto a cutting board and cut it with a sharp knife into ½-inch-thick slices. Lightly spray a large nonstick skillet with vegetable oil cooking spray and place it over medium-high heat. Arrange polenta slices in a single layer about 1 inch apart and cook 5 minutes. Turn and cook second side 5 minutes. Repeat with remaining polenta.

> Per 1-cup serving: 110 calories; 2 g protein; 23 g carbohydrate;
> 2 g fiber; 1 g fat; 592 mg sodium; calories from protein: 9%;
> calories from carbohydrates: 82%; calories from fats: 9%

• • •

Quinoa

MAKES 3 1-CUP SERVINGS

Quinoa ("keen-wah") comes from the high plains of the Andes Mountains, where it is nicknamed "the mother grain" for its life-giving properties. The National Academy of Sciences has called quinoa "one of the best sources of protein in the vegetable kingdom," because of its excellent amino acid pattern. Quinoa cooks quickly, and as it cooks the germ unfolds like a little tail. It has a light, fluffy texture, and may be eaten plain, used as a pilaf, or as an addition to soups and stews. The dry grain is coated with a bitter-tasting substance called saponin, which repels insects and birds and protects it from ultraviolet radiation. Quinoa must be washed thoroughly before cooking to remove this bitter coating. The easiest way to wash it is to place it in a strainer and rinse it with cool water until the water runs clear.

1 cup quinoa	2 cups boiling water

Rinse quinoa thoroughly in a fine sieve, then add it to boiling water in a saucepan. Reduce to a simmer, then cover loosely and cook until quinoa is tender and fluffy, about 15 minutes.

Per 1-cup serving: 212 calories; 8 g protein; 40 g carbohydrate;
4 g fat; 4 g fiber; 12 mg sodium; calories from protein: 14%;
calories from carbohydrates: 72%; calories from fats: 14%

● ● ●

Ginger Noodles

MAKES 4 1-CUP SERVINGS

These exotic-tasting noodles are surprisingly easy to prepare. Soba noodles are made from buckwheat flour and are sold in natural food stores and Asian markets.

1 8-ounce package soba noodles	2 garlic cloves, minced
3 tablespoons seasoned rice vinegar	½ to 1 jalapeño pepper, finely chopped
3 tablespoons reduced-sodium soy sauce	2 green onions, finely chopped, including tops
2 teaspoons finely chopped fresh ginger	¼ cup chopped fresh cilantro (optional)

Cook noodles in boiling water according to package directions. When tender, drain and rinse.

Mix vinegar, soy sauce, ginger, garlic, pepper, onions, and cilantro (if using). Pour over cooked noodles and toss to mix.

Per 1-cup serving: 184 calories; 10 g protein; 40 g carbohydrate;
0.2 g fat; 2 g fiber; 914 mg sodium; calories from protein: 20%;
calories from carbohydrates: 79%; calories from fats: 1%

• • •

Kasha with Cabbage

MAKES ABOUT 5 ½-CUP SERVINGS

Toasted buckwheat groats are known as "kasha" and have a distinctive hearty flavor that goes well with cooked cabbage. Look for kasha in natural food stores and some supermarkets.

2 teaspoons olive oil
½ cup kasha
2 cups finely chopped cabbage

1 cup vegetable broth or water
¼ teaspoon salt

Heat oil in a large saucepan. Add kasha and shredded cabbage and cook over medium high heat, stirring constantly, for 1 minute.

Stir in vegetable broth and salt. Cover and simmer until kasha is tender and all the liquid is absorbed, about 10 minutes.

Per ½-cup serving: 45 calories; 1.5 g protein; 6 g carbohydrate;
2 g fat; 1 g fiber; 206 mg sodium; calories from protein:
12%; calories from carbohydrates: 48%; calories from fats: 40%

SANDWICHES AND WRAPS

Baked Tofu Sandwich

MAKES 2 SANDWICHES

Baked tofu makes a wonderful snack or sandwich filling. It is firm and flavorful and comes in a variety of flavors. Look for it in the deli case at your natural food store or supermarket.

1 package baked tofu
4 slices whole wheat or rye bread
1 to 2 tablespoons stone-ground
mustard

1 to 2 tablespoons Tofu Mayo
(page 173) or vegan mayonnaise
6 lettuce leaves
6 tomato slices

Cut tofu into ⅛-inch-thick slices.

Spread bread lightly with mustard and Tofu Mayo. Top with slices of tofu, lettuce, and tomato.

Per sandwich: 255 calories; 14 g protein; 38 g carbohydrate;
7 g fat; 6 g fiber; 439 mg sodium; calories from protein: 20%;
calories from carbohydrates: 56%; calories from fats: 24%

• • •

Teriyaki Spice Baked Tofu
MAKES 6 ¼-INCH-THICK SLICES

The firm texture and delicious flavor of baked tofu makes it perfect as a snack, sandwich filling, or stir-fry ingredient. Begin with tofu that is firm enough to spring back when lightly pressed. If it fails this test, begin by pressing it as directed below.

1 pound firm fresh tofu	1 garlic clove crushed
2 tablespoons apple juice concen- trate	¼ teaspoon powdered ginger or ½ teaspoon minced fresh ginger
3 tablespoons reduced-sodium soy sauce	scant pinch cayenne pepper, or more to taste

To press tofu if necessary: Line a baking sheet with a clean dish towel. Cut tofu into 6 slices, each about ¼-inch thick, and place on the towel in a single layer. Cover with a second clean dish towel, and top with a cutting board. Place several heavy objects (canned food, books, jars of beans) on the cutting board. Let stand 30 minutes.

In the meantime, prepare the marinade. Combine apple juice concentrate, soy sauce, garlic, ginger, and cayenne pepper in a small measuring cup or mixing bowl.

Remove tofu from the press and pat dry. Carefully arrange the slices in a sandwich-size zip-top plastic bag, then add marinade. Seal the bag then carefully massage it so that all the tofu slices are coated with marinade. Refrigerate 4 hours or more (overnight is ideal), turning the bag occasionally to keep all the slices coated.

Preheat oven to 375°F.

Remove tofu from the bag and place it in one layer in a glass baking dish. Drizzle with any remaining marinade. Bake, uncovered, until dry and deep golden brown, about 35 minutes.

Per slice: 75 calories; 7 g protein; 5 g carbohydrate; 4 g fat;
1 g fiber; 259 mg sodium; calories from protein: 34%;
calories from carbohydrates: 25%; calories from fats: 41%

• • •

Bean Burgers
MAKES 6 BURGERS

These burgers make a great summer meal with potato salad, corn on the cob, and watermelon.

1   cup cooked garbanzo beans
1   cup cooked Brown Rice (page 157)
½ cup quick-cooking rolled oats
1   stalk celery, finely chopped
1   small onion, finely chopped
1   garlic clove, minced
2   tablespoons reduced-sodium soy sauce
1   teaspoon paprika
¼ teaspoon black pepper
6   whole wheat burger buns
6   tablespoons Tofu Mayo (page 173) or other vegan mayonnaise
6   tablespoons stone-ground mustard
6   tablespoons ketchup
6   lettuce leaves
6   tomato slices
6   red onion slices

Drain garbanzo beans and mash coarsely. Mix with brown rice, oats, celery, onion, garlic, soy sauce, paprika, and black pepper.

Form into six patties. Cook in an oil-sprayed nonstick skillet over medium heat until lightly browned on both sides.

Warm the buns, then spread with one tablespoon each Tofu Mayo, mustard, and ketchup. Place a burger patty topped with a tomato slice, onion slice, and lettuce leaf on each bun.

Per burger: 334 calories; 14 g protein; 62 g carbohydrate;
6 g fat; 8 g fiber; 552 mg sodium; calories from protein: 16%;
calories from carbohydrates: 70%; calories from fats: 14%

• • •

Zucchini Pockets
MAKES 8 SANDWICHES

2   medium zucchini, thinly sliced (2 to 3 cups)
1   tomato, diced (about 1 cup)
2   vegan burger patties, crumbled (see box, page 165)
1   teaspoon reduced-sodium soy sauce
¼ teaspoon basil
¼ teaspoon oregano
¼ teaspoon garlic powder
¼ teaspoon black pepper
4   pieces whole wheat pita bread

Combine zucchini, tomato, crumbled burger patties, soy sauce, basil, oregano, garlic powder, and black pepper in a large nonstick skillet.

Cover and cook over medium heat, stirring often, until zucchini is tender, about 5 minutes.

Warm a pita bread by placing it in a vegetable steamer over boiling water for about 30 seconds. Cut in half and stuff with zucchini mixture. Repeat with remaining pitas.

Per pocket: 103 calories; 8 g protein; 17 g carbohydrate;
0.7 g fat; 4 g fiber; 167 mg sodium; calories from protein: 30%;
calories from carbohydrates: 63%; calories from fats: 7%

Meatlike Sandwiches, Burgers, and Hot Dogs

A wide variety of meatless cold cuts, burgers, and hot dogs are sold in natural food stores and most supermarkets. A sampling of these products is shown below. Check the deli case as well as the freezer section for these products and others. Be sure to read the ingredient list to determine that there are no animal ingredients, such as eggs, egg whites, cheese, whey, or casein. Check the nutritional information as well to determine the amounts of fat and sodium.

MEATLESS COLD CUTS AND DELI SLICES

Smart Bacon (Lightlife Foods)
Foney Baloney (Lightlife Foods)
Smart Deli Turkey (Lightlife Foods)
Smart Deli Bologna (Lightlife Foods)
Smart Deli Ham (Lightlife Foods)
Soylami (Lightlife Foods)
Pepperoni (Lightlife Foods)
Lean Links Sausage (Lightlife Foods)
Veggie Bologna Slices (Yves Fine Foods)
Veggie Pizza Pepperoni Slices (Yves Fine Foods)
Veggie Ham Slices (Yves Fine Foods)
Veggie Turkey Slices (Yves Fine Foods)
Veggie Salami Slices (Yves Fine Foods)

MEATLESS BURGERS

Veggie Cuisine Burger (Yves Fine Foods)
Veggie Burger Burgers (Yves Fine Foods)

Garden Vegetable Patties (Yves Fine Foods)
Black Bean and Mushroom Burgers (Yves Fine Foods)
Veggie Chick'n Burger (Yves Fine Foods)
LightBurgers (Lightlife Foods)
Prime Burger (White Wave Inc.)
Green Giant Harvest Burger (Pillsbury Company)
Vegan Original Boca Burger (Boca Burger Company)
Superburgers (Turtle Island Foods)
Natural Touch Vegan Burger (Worthington Foods)
Garden Vegan Burger (Wholesome and Hearty Foods)
Gardenburger Hamburger Style (Wholesome and Hearty Foods)
Amy's California Veggie Burger (Amy's Kitchen)
Amy's All American Burger (Amy's Kitchen)
Soy Deli All Natural Tofu Burger (Qwong Hop & Company)

MEATLESS HOT DOGS

Veggie Dogs (Yves Fine Foods)
Jumbo Veggie Dogs (Yves Fine Foods)
Hot & Spicy Jumbo Veggie Dogs (Yves Fine Foods)
Good Dogs (Yves Fine Foods)
Tofu Dogs (Yves Fine Foods)
Smart Dogs (Lightlife Foods)
Wild Dogs (Wildwood Natural Foods)

OTHER MEATLESS PRODUCTS

Smart Ground (Lightlife Foods)
Veggie Ground Round Original (Yves Fine Foods)
Veggie Ground Round Italian (Yves Fine Foods)
Veggie Breakfast Links (Yves Fine Foods)
Canadian Veggie Bacon (Yves Fine Foods)
Veggie Breakfast Patties (Yves Fine Foods)
Chiken Chunks (Harvest Direct)
Chiken Breasts (Harvest Direct)
Tofurky Deli Slices (Turtle Island Foods)
Tofurky Jerky (Turtle Island Foods)
Not Chicken Deli Slices (United Specialty Foods)
White Wave Sandwich Slices (White Wave Foods)

Thai Wrap

Thai Wraps make it easy to increase your intake of healthful, protective vegetables.

1 tablespoon peanut butter	1½ teaspoons curry powder
2 tablespoons reduced-sodium soy sauce	½ red bell pepper, diced
1 small onion, chopped	½ cup chopped cilantro (optional)
1 carrot, thinly sliced	2 cups finely chopped kale
1 celery stalk, thinly sliced	8 large flour tortillas
2 cups sliced mushrooms (about ½ pound)	6 tablespoons Apple Chutney (page 177)
½ pound firm tofu, cut into ½-inch cubes (about 1 cup)	

Mix peanut butter with 3 tablespoons water. Set aside.

Heat ½ cup water and soy sauce in a large nonstick skillet. Add onion, carrot, celery, and mushrooms. Cook 5 minutes, stirring occasionally.

Stir in tofu and cook over medium-high heat, stirring often, until vegetables are tender, about 5 minutes.

Stir in curry powder, pepper, cilantro, kale, and peanut butter mixture. Cover and cook until kale is tender, about 5 minutes.

Heat tortillas in a dry skillet until soft. Top each with about ½ cup of the vegetable mixture and 2 teaspoons Apple Chutney. Roll tortilla around filling.

Per wrap: 207 calories; 8 g protein; 35 g carbohydrate; 5 g fat;
3 g fiber; 461 mg sodium; calories from protein: 15%;
calories from carbohydrates: 65%; calories from fats: 20%

● ● ●

Broccoli Burritos

You'll love broccoli, the powerful protector, rolled in a flour tortilla with a tangy garbanzo spread. Roasted red peppers are sold in supermarkets, usually near the pickles. Sesame butter, also called tahini ("ta-hee-nee"), is sold in natural food stores, ethnic markets, and many supermarkets. Look for it near the peanut butter, or in the ethnic food section.

2 or 3 stalks of broccoli
1   15-ounce can garbanzo beans
½ cup roasted red peppers
2   tablespoons tahini

3   tablespoons lemon juice
6   flour tortillas
6   tablespoons salsa, or more to
     taste

Cut or break broccoli into florets. Peel stalks and cut into ½-inch-thick rounds. Steam over boiling water until just barely tender, about 5 minutes.

Drain garbanzo beans and place in a food processor with peppers, tahini, and lemon juice. Process until completely smooth, about 2 minutes. Spread about ¼ cup of the garbanzo mixture on a tortilla and place in a large heated skillet. Heat until tortilla is warm and soft, about 2 minutes. Arrange a line of cooked broccoli down the center, then sprinkle with salsa. Roll tortilla around filling. Repeat with remaining tortillas.

Per burrito: 199 calories; 8 g protein; 31 g carbohydrate;
6 g fat; 4 g fiber; 225 mg sodium; calories from protein: 16%;
calories from carbohydrates: 60%; calories from fats: 24%

• • •

Middle Eastern Roll-ups
MAKES 6 TO 8 ROLL-UPS

These roll-ups are a complete meal in an edible wrapper. Easily portable, they are perfect for lunches or picnics. The garbanzo spread can be prepared in a food processor or by hand. Directions for both methods are given.

2   garlic cloves
1   15-ounce can of garbanzo beans
2   tablespoons tahini (sesame
     butter)
2   tablespoons lemon juice
¼ teaspoon cumin
¼ teaspoon paprika

2   cups cooked Brown Rice (see
     page 157)
6 to 8 flour tortillas or chapatis
3   cups (approximately) mixed
     salad greens or torn leaf lettuce
1   cup chopped green onions
1   cup chopped cilantro (optional)

Place garlic in a food processor and chop finely.

Drain beans, reserving liquid, then add them to the food processor along with tahini, lemon juice, cumin, and paprika. Process until smooth and spreadable. If mixture is too dry, add some of the reserved bean liquid to achieve a spreadable consistency.

To prepare filling by hand: drain beans, reserving liquid, and mash until very smooth. Crush garlic and add to beans, along with tahini, lemon juice, cumin, paprika, and salt. Mix well. Thin to a spreadable consistency with reserved bean liquid if needed.

Warm a tortilla in a large dry skillet, flipping to warm both sides until soft and pliable. Remove from pan and spread evenly to within an inch of the edge with about ½ cup of garbanzo mixture.

Top with ¼ to ½ cup brown rice. Add salad greens, green onions, and chopped cilantro if using. Wrap tortilla around filling. Repeat with remaining tortillas.

Per roll-up: 256 calories; 10 g protein; 43 g carbohydrate;
6 g fat; 4 g fiber; 236 mg sodium; calories from protein: 15%;
calories from carbohydrates: 65%; calories from fats: 20%

SALADS

Fresh Broccoli Salad
MAKES ABOUT 4 1-CUP SERVINGS

Enjoy the great flavor and protective power of tender crisp broccoli in this delicious salad. Toasted sesame oil, available in Asian markets and large grocery stores, gives the salad its aroma and distinctive flavor.

1 bunch broccoli	½ cup seasoned rice vinegar
1 medium red onion, finely sliced	1 tablespoon toasted sesame oil
1 or 2 garlic cloves, minced	½ teaspoon dried red pepper flakes

Cut or break broccoli into small florets. Transfer to a salad bowl. Add remaining ingredients and toss to mix. Chill, tossing once or twice, for 20 minutes or longer before serving.

Per 1-cup serving: 64 calories; 2 g protein; 6 g carbohydrate;
4 g fat; 3 g fiber; 620 mg sodium; calories from protein: 16%;
calories from carbohydrates: 38%; calories from fats: 46%

● ● ●

Fresh Tomatoes with Basil
MAKES ABOUT 6 SERVINGS

This beautiful salad is one of the best ways to enjoy juicy vine-ripened tomatoes of summertime.

2 or 3 ripe red tomatoes	¼ cup chopped fresh basil
¼ cup thinly sliced sweet onion (such as Vidalia, Walla Walla, or Maui)	2 teaspoons balsamic vinegar freshly ground black pepper

Slice tomatoes and put them in a serving dish, with the onion and basil. Sprinkle with vinegar and freshly ground black pepper and toss gently to mix.

Per serving: 27 calories; 1 g protein; 6 g carbohydrate; 03 g fat;
1 g fiber; 9 mg sodium; calories from protein: 13%;
calories from carbohydrates: 77%; calories from fats: 10%

• • •

Tex-Mex Salad

MAKES 6 ½-CUP SERVINGS

Serve this colorful salad with whole wheat bread or roll it up in a whole wheat tortilla. The jalapeño pepper is quite hot and should be handled with care. It can be omitted if you prefer a milder salad.

1   15-ounce can black-eyed peas
1   red or yellow bell pepper, seeded and diced
1   small jalapeño pepper, finely chopped (more or less to taste)
½ cup chopped green onions
1   tomato, diced
¼ cup chopped fresh cilantro (optional)
1   garlic clove, pressed or minced
¼ cup seasoned rice vinegar
1   teaspoon ground cumin

Drain peas and combine with peppers, green onions, tomato, cilantro, garlic, vinegar, and cumin in a large bowl. Toss gently to mix. If time permits, chill 1 to 2 hours before serving.

Per ½-cup serving: 82 calories; 3 g protein; 18 g carbohydrate;
0.4 g fat; 4 g fiber; 363 mg sodium; calories from protein: 14%;
calories from carbohydrates: 82%; calories from fats: 4%

• • •

Watermelon Salad

MAKES 3 1-CUP SERVINGS

Does watermelon and onions in the same dish sound a little unusual? Take my word for it, the combination is wonderful! This recipe was created by Jean Marc Fulsack, chef for Dr. Dean Ornish's lifestyle-change program.

3   cups seedless watermelon cubes
¼ cup finely chopped red onion, rinsed
2   tablespoons balsamic vinegar
1   tablespoon seasoned rice vinegar
2   tablespoons fresh mint, finely chopped, or ½ teaspoon dried mint
¼ teaspoon freshly ground black pepper

Combine watermelon and onion in a salad bowl. Whisk together vinegars, mint, and pepper. Pour over watermelon and toss gently to mix. If possible, chill before serving.

Per 1-cup serving: 73 calories; 1 g protein; 17 g carbohydrate; 0.7 g fat; 0.5 g fiber; 183 mg sodium; calories from protein: 6%; calories from carbohydrates: 86%; calories from fats: 8%

• • •

Mixed Greens with Apples and Walnuts
MAKES ABOUT 7 1-CUP SERVINGS

This simple salad is especially delicious in the autumn when apples are fresh. Using a prewashed salad mix makes it easy to prepare.

6 cups salad mix, or washed and torn butter lettuce
1 tart green apple (Granny Smith, pippin, or similar), cored and diced

¼ cup chopped walnuts
3 to 4 tablespoons seasoned rice vinegar

Place salad mix or torn lettuce in a bowl. Add apple and walnuts. Sprinkle with seasoned rice vinegar and toss to mix.

Per 1-cup serving: 31 calories; 1 g protein; 4 g carbohydrate; 2 g fat; 1 g fiber; 141 mg sodium; calories from protein: 10%; calories from carbohydrates: 46%; calories from fats: 44%

• • •

Red Potato Salad
MAKES ABOUT 6 1-CUP SERVINGS

4 large red potatoes, scrubbed
½ cup thinly sliced red onion
1 red or yellow bell pepper, seeded and sliced
¼ cup finely chopped fresh parsley
¼ cup cider vinegar
2 tablespoons seasoned rice vinegar

juice of 1 lemon
2 garlic cloves, pressed
2 teaspoons stone-ground mustard
½ teaspoon salt
¼ to ½ teaspoon black pepper

Cut potatoes into ½-inch cubes and steam over boiling water until just tender, 10 to 15 minutes. Rinse with cold water, then transfer to a large bowl. Add red onion, bell pepper, and parsley.

Combine vinegars, lemon juice, garlic, mustard, salt, and pepper. Pour over salad. Toss to mix.

Per 1-cup serving: 164 calories; 4 g protein; 38 g carbohydrate;
0.4 g fat; 4 g fiber; 410 mg sodium; calories from protein: 9%;
calories from carbohydrates: 89%; calories from fats: 2%

• • •

Carrot, Beet, and Jicama Salad
MAKES ABOUT 8 ½-CUP SERVINGS

Three colorful root vegetables combine to make a crunchy, nutritious salad.

2 or 3 medium beets	3 tablespoons lemon juice
1 small jicama, peeled and cut in thin strips or diced	2 tablespoons seasoned rice vinegar
2 carrots, peeled and cut in thin strips or diced	2 teaspoons stone-ground mustard
	½ teaspoon dill weed

Cut stems and roots off beets, then steam until tender, about 20 minutes. When cool enough to handle, slip skins off. Cut beets into ½-inch cubes and put in a salad bowl. Add jicama and carrots.

Mix lemon juice, vinegar, mustard, and dill. Pour over salad. Toss to mix. If time permits, chill before serving.

Per ½-cup serving: 30 calories; 1 g protein; 7 g carbohydrate;
0.2 g fat; 2 g fiber; 187 mg sodium; calories from protein: 10%;
calories from carbohydrates: 84%; calories from fats: 6%

• • •

Spinach Salad with Orange Sesame Dressing
MAKES ABOUT 6 1-CUP SERVINGS

Toasted sesame seeds add wonderful flavor to this salad.

1 5 cups fresh spinach leaves	2 tablespoons seasoned rice vinegar
1 red or yellow bell pepper, seeded and cut into strips	1 tablespoon orange juice concentrate
½ cup thinly sliced red onion	1 tablespoon water
1 navel orange	
1 tablespoon sesame seeds	

Trim off spinach stems. Carefully wash the leaves, dry them, then tear any large leaves into bite-size pieces. Place in a salad bowl along with pepper and onion.

Peel the orange, then cut it in half from top to bottom. Slice each half into thin half circles and add to the salad.

Spread sesame seeds out on pan and toast in a 400°F toaster oven (or regular oven) for 10 minutes. Transfer to a blender and grind into a powder. Mix with vinegar, orange juice concentrate, and water. Pour over salad and toss just before serving.

Per 1-cup serving: 48 calories; 2.1 g protein; 9 g carbohydrate;
0.8 g fat; 2 g fiber; 185 mg sodium; calories from protein: 16%;
calories from carbohydrates: 70%; calories from fats: 14%

DIPS, DRESSINGS, AND SAUCES

Black Bean Dip
MAKES ABOUT 2 CUPS

Serve this dip with baked tortilla chips or use it as a burrito filling. You'll find instant black bean flakes (see Glossary) in natural food stores and some supermarkets.

1 cup instant black bean flakes	½ to 1 cup salsa (you choose the
1 cup boiling water	heat)

Mix bean flakes and boiling water. Let stand 5 minutes. Stir in salsa to taste.

Per ¼-cup serving: 63 calories; 4 g protein; 12 g carbohydrate;
0.2 g fat; 4 g fiber; 117 mg sodium; calories from protein: 25%;
calories from carbohydrates: 72%; calories from fats: 3%

● ● ●

Corn Butter
MAKES ABOUT 2 CUPS

This creamy yellow spread is a low-fat alternative to margarine. Emes Jel and agar powder are thickening agents that are sold in natural food stores.

¼ cup cornmeal	½ teaspoon salt
2 teaspoons Emes Jel (see Glossary) or 1½ teaspoons agar powder	2 teaspoons lemon juice
	1 tablespoon finely grated raw carrot
1 cup boiling water	1 teaspoon nutritional yeast
2 tablespoons raw cashews	(optional)

Combine cornmeal with 1 cup water in a small saucepan. Simmer, stirring frequently, until very thick, about 10 minutes. Set aside.

Combine Emes Jel or agar powder with ¼ cup cold water in a blender. Let stand at least 3 minutes. Add 1 cup boiling water and blend to mix. Add cooked cornmeal, cashews, salt, lemon juice, grated carrot, and yeast, if using. Cover and blend until totally smooth (this is essential and will take several minutes). Transfer to a covered container and chill until thickened, 2 to 3 hours.

> Per tablespoon: 7 calories; 0.2 g protein; 1 g carbohydrate;
> 0.2 g fat; 0.1 g fiber; 34 mg sodium; calories from protein: 11%;
> calories from carbohydrates: 57%; calories from fats: 32%

• • •

Brown Gravy
MAKES ABOUT 2 CUPS

This traditional-tasting gravy is low in fat and delicious on potatoes, rice, or vegetables.

2 cups water or vegetable broth	2 tablespoons cornstarch
1 tablespoon cashews	3 tablespoons reduced-sodium soy sauce
1 tablespoon onion powder	
½ teaspoon garlic granules or powder	

Combine all ingredients in blender container. Blend until completely smooth, 2 to 3 minutes.

Transfer to a saucepan and cook over medium heat, stirring constantly, until thickened.

> Per ¼-cup serving: 23 calories; 1 g protein; 4 g carbohydrate;
> 0.5 g fat; 0.1 g fiber; 190 mg sodium; calories from protein: 15%;
> calories from carbohydrates: 65%; calories from fats: 20%

• • •

Tofu Mayo
MAKES ABOUT 1½ CUPS

Use this low-fat mayonnaise substitute on sandwiches and salads.

1 12.3-ounce package Mori-Nu Lite Silken Tofu (firm or extra firm)	1 teaspoon Dijon mustard
¾ teaspoon salt	1½ tablespoons lemon juice
½ teaspoon sugar	1½ tablespoons seasoned rice vinegar

Combine tofu, salt, sugar, mustard, lemon juice and vinegar in a food processor or blender, and process until completely smooth, 1 to 2 minutes. Chill thoroughly before using.

Per tablespoon: 6 calories; 1 g protein; 0.4 g carbohydrate;
0.1 g fat; 0 g fiber; 93 mg sodium; calories from protein: 48%;
calories from carbohydrates: 29%; calories from fats: 23%

• • •

Salsa Fresca

MAKES ABOUT 6 CUPS

This fresh and chunky salsa is quite mild. For a hotter salsa, increase the jalapeños or red pepper flakes.

4   large ripe tomatoes, chopped
    (about 4 cups)
1   small onion, finely chopped
1   bell pepper, finely chopped
1   jalapeño pepper, seeded and
    finely chopped, or 1 teaspoon
    red pepper flakes

4   garlic cloves, minced
1   cup chopped cilantro leaves
1   15-ounce can tomato sauce
2   tablespoons cider vinegar
1½ teaspoons cumin

Combine all ingredients in a mixing bowl. Stir to mix. Let stand 1 hour before serving.

Note: Salsa will keep in the refrigerator for about 2 weeks. It also freezes well.

Per tablespoon: 4 calories; 0.1 g protein; 1 g carbohydrate;
0.03 g fat; 0.2 g fiber; 27 mg sodium; calories from protein: 14%;
calories from carbohydrates: 79%; calories from fats: 7%

• • •

Sesame Salt

MAKES ½ CUP

Sesame Salt is a delicious alternative to butter or margarine on cooked grains, baked potatoes, or steamed vegetables. Unhulled sesame seeds (sometimes called "brown sesame seeds") are sold in natural food stores and some supermarkets.

½ cup unhulled sesame seeds   ½ teaspoon salt

Toast sesame seeds in a dry skillet over medium heat, stirring constantly until they begin to pop and brown slightly, about 5 minutes. Transfer to a blender. Add salt and grind into a uniform powder. Transfer to an airtight container. Store in refrigerator.

> Per tablespoon: 52 calories; 2 g protein; 2 g carbohydrate;
> 4 g fat; 1 g fiber; 134 mg sodium; calories from protein: 12%;
> calories from carbohydrates: 15%; calories from fats: 73%

● ● ●

Sesame Seasoning
MAKES ½ CUP

Sesame Seasoning is delicious with steamed vegetables, cooked grains, and legumes. Unhulled sesame seeds are light brown in color and are sold in natural food stores and some supermarkets.

½ cup unhulled sesame seeds   2 tablespoons nutritional yeast
½ teaspoon salt

Toast sesame seeds in a dry skillet over medium heat. Stir constantly until seeds begin to pop and brown slightly, about 5 minutes.

Transfer to a blender, add salt and nutritional yeast and grind into a fine powder.

Transfer to an airtight container. Store in refrigerator.

> Per tablespoon: 57 calories; 2 g protein; 3 g carbohydrate;
> 4 g fat; 1 g fiber; 137 mg sodium; calories from protein: 15%;
> calories from carbohydrates: 19%; calories from fats: 66%

● ● ●

Simple Vinaigrette
MAKES ½ CUP

Seasoned rice vinegar makes a delicious salad dressing all by itself, or enhanced with mustard and garlic.

½ cup seasoned rice vinegar   1 clove garlic, pressed
1 to 2 teaspoons stone-ground or
   Dijon-style mustard

Whisk all ingredients together. Use as a dressing for salads and for steamed vegetables.

> Per tablespoon: 27 calories; 0.1 g protein; 6 g carbohydrate;
> 0.1 g fat; 0 g fiber; 562 mg sodium; calories from protein: 2%;
> calories from carbohydrates: 94%; calories from fats: 4%

● ● ●

Balsamic Vinaigrette

Makes ¼ cup

The mellow flavor of balsamic vinegar is delicious on salads.

2 tablespoons balsamic vinegar
2 tablespoons seasoned rice vinegar

1 tablespoon ketchup
1 teaspoon stone-ground mustard
1 garlic clove, pressed

Whisk vinegars, ketchup, mustard, and garlic together.

Per tablespoon: 20 calories; 0.1 g protein; 4.5 g carbohydrate;
0.08 g fat; 0.05 g fiber; 229 mg sodium; calories from protein: 3%;
calories from carbohydrates: 93%; calories from fats: 4%

• • •

Raspberry or Blackberry Vinaigrette

Makes ¼ cup

This dressing adds a delightful fruity taste to salads.

2 tablespoons raspberry or black-berry vinegar

2 tablespoons seasoned rice vinegar

Whisk vinegars together.

Per tablespoon: 11 calories; 0.04 g protein; 2.5 g carbohydrate;
0 g fat; 0 g fiber; 268 mg sodium; calories from protein: 2%;
calories from carbohydrates: 98%; calories from fats: 0%

• • •

Liquid Gold Dressing

Makes 2 cups

Vesanto Melina, R.D., developed this dressing for use on salads, baked potatoes, rice, steamed broccoli, and other veggies. She gave it the name "Liquid Gold," not just because of the color and delicious flavor, but because of its nutritional value. Two tablespoons provides 3.8 g of omega-3 fatty acids (your day's supply, and then some) along with 40 percent of your B_{12} for the day (80 percent if you use the higher amount of yeast powder). In addition, this creamy dressing is packed with riboflavin and other B vitamins.

½ cup flaxseed oil
½ cup water
⅓ cup lemon juice
2   tablespoons balsamic or rasp-
     berry vinegar
¼ cup Bragg Liquid Aminos or
     tamari soy sauce

¼ to ½ cup nutritional yeast
     powder or flakes
2   teaspoons Dijon mustard
1   teaspoon cumin

Combine all ingredients in blender container. Blend until smooth.
Dressing can be kept in a jar with lid, refrigerated for two weeks.

Per tablespoon: 39 calories; 0.5 g protein; 1 g carbohydrate;
3.5 g fat; 0.2 g fiber; 90 mg sodium; calories from protein: 7%;
calories from carbohydrate: 8%; calories from fat: 85%

● ● ●

Creamy Dill Dressing
MAKES ABOUT 1½ CUPS

*This rich-tasting, creamy dressing has no added oil. Its creaminess comes
from tofu.*

1   12.3-ounce package Mori-Nu
     firm tofu
2   tablespoons lemon juice
3   tablespoons seasoned rice
     vinegar

1   tablespoon cider vinegar
1   teaspoon garlic granules or
     powder
½ teaspoon dill weed
¼ teaspoon salt

Combine all ingredients in a food processor or blender. Blend until completely smooth, 1 to 2 minutes. Store any extra dressing in an airtight
container in the refrigerator.

Per tablespoon: 12 calories; 1 g protein; 1 g carbohydrate; 1 g fat;
0.1 g fiber; 90 mg sodium; calories from protein: 36%;
calories from carbohydrates: 18%; calories from fats: 46%

● ● ●

Apple Chutney
MAKES ABOUT 4 CUPS

*Chutney is a spicy relish served as a condiment with Indian meals. This
basic chutney will keep in the refrigerator for several weeks, and may be
frozen for longer storage.*

3 large tart green apples (Granny
   Smith, pippin, or similar)
1 cup cider vinegar
1 cup sugar or other sweetener
1 large garlic clove, minced
1 tablespoon minced ginger root
   or ½ teaspoon powdered ginger

½ cup orange juice
1 teaspoon cinnamon
1 teaspoon powdered cloves
½ teaspoon salt
¼ teaspoon cayenne, or more to
   taste

Core apples and chop coarsely. Combine with vinegar, sugar, garlic, ginger root, orange juice, cinnamon, cloves, salt, and cayenne in a sauce pan.

Bring to a slow simmer and cook uncovered, stirring occasionally, until most of the liquid is absorbed, about 1 hour.

Per tablespoon: 22 calories; 0.1 g protein; 6 g carbohydrate;
0.04 g fat; 0.2 g fiber; 17 mg sodium; calories from protein: 1%;
calories from carbohydrates: 97%; calories from fats: 2%

• • •

Cranberry Persimmon Relish
MAKES ABOUT 2 CUPS

Cranberries and fuyu persimmons make a colorful autumn relish in which the sweetness of the persimmons is a perfect foil for the tart cranberries. Fuyu persimmons, which are eaten while still crisp, are sold in many supermarkets and natural food stores.

2 fuyu persimmons
1 cup cranberries, fresh or frozen
2 tablespoons orange juice
   concentrate

1 tablespoon sugar or other
   sweetener
½ teaspoon powdered ginger

Remove stems, then coarsely chop persimmons in a food processor. Add cranberries, orange juice concentrate, sugar, and ginger. Process using quick pulses until coarsely and uniformly chopped. Let stand 20 minutes before serving.

Per ¼-cup serving: 49 calories; 0.5 g protein; 13 g carbohydrate;
0.1 g fat; 2 g fiber; 0.5 mg sodium; calories from protein: 3%;
calories from carbohydrates: 95%; calories from fats: 2%

• • •

Blueberry Sauce

MAKES ABOUT 3 CUPS

Use this colorful sauce as a spread on bread or toast or as a dessert topping. Agar is a thickener made from a sea vegetable that can be used in place of animal gelatin. It is sold in natural food stores and Asian markets.

1 cup apple juice concentrate	1½ teaspoons agar powder
3 cups fresh blueberries or 1 16-ounce bag frozen blueberries	1 tablespoon lemon juice

In a blender, combine 1 cup water with apple juice concentrate, 2 cups of the blueberries, and the agar powder. Blend until fairly smooth.

Transfer mixture to a saucepan and simmer, stirring occasionally, for 3 minutes. Remove from heat. Add remaining berries and the lemon juice. Stir to mix. Chill thoroughly, 3 to 4 hours.

Per tablespoon: 15 calories; 0.09 g protein; 4 g carbohydrate;
0.06 g fat; 0.2 g fiber; 2 mg sodium; calories from protein: 3%;
calories from carbohydrates: 94%; calories from fats: 3%

● ● ●

Pineapple Apricot Sauce

MAKES ABOUT 3 CUPS

Use this sauce as a spread on toast or as a topping for cake. It is delicious with Quick and Easy Brown Bread (page 207). It is thickened with agar, a sea vegetable thickener that is sold in natural food stores and Asian markets.

1 cup apple juice concentrate	1 8-ounce can crushed pineapple, packed in pineapple juice
1½ teaspoons agar powder	
1 cup chopped apricots, fresh, frozen, or canned	¼ teaspoon ginger

Combine apple juice and agar with 1 cup water in a saucepan. Let stand 5 minutes. Bring to a simmer, stirring occasionally, and cook 3 minutes.

Add apricots, pineapple with its juice, and ginger. Stir to mix. Remove from heat and chill thoroughly, 3 to 4 hours.

Per tablespoon: 13 calories; 0.08 g protein; 3 g carbohydrate;
0 .05 g fat; 0.1 g fiber; 2 mg sodium; calories from protein: 3%;
calories from carbohydrates: 94%; calories from fats: 3%

SOUPS AND STEWS

Vegetable Broth

MAKES ABOUT 2 QUARTS

A steamy cup of this broth makes a warm and comforting meal. It may also be used as an ingredient in recipes that call for broth or stock.

1 onion, chopped	¼ teaspoon turmeric
1 carrot, chopped	¼ teaspoon garlic powder
1 celery stalk, chopped	¼ teaspoon marjoram
¼ cup chopped fresh parsley	½ teaspoon salt
6 cups water	1 15-ounce can garbanzo beans,
2 teaspoons onion powder	including liquid
½ teaspoon thyme	

Combine onion, carrot, celery, parsley, water, onion powder, thyme, turmeric, garlic powder, and marjoram in a large pot. Cover and simmer 20 minutes.

Stir in garbanzo beans with their liquid. Transfer to a blender in small batches and process until completely smooth, about 1 minute per batch. Be sure to hold the lid on tightly and start the blender on the lowest speed.

Per 1-cup serving: 80 calories; 3 g protein; 16 g carbohydrate;
1 g fat; 3 g fiber; 302 mg sodium; calories from protein: 15%;
calories from carbohydrates: 77%; calories from fats: 8%

• • •

Green Velvet Soup

MAKES ABOUT 2½ QUARTS (10 1-CUP SERVINGS)

This beautiful soup provides an abundance of nourishing green vegetables.

1 onion, chopped	2 medium stalks broccoli,
2 celery stalks, sliced	chopped
2 potatoes, scrubbed and diced	1 6-ounce bag prewashed spinach
¾ cup split peas, rinsed	½ teaspoon basil
2 bay leaves	¼ teaspoon black pepper
6 cups water or vegetable broth	½ to 1 teaspoon salt
1 medium zucchini, diced	

Place onion, celery, potatoes, split peas, and bay leaves in a large pot. Add water or broth and bring to a simmer. Cover and cook until peas are tender, about 45 minutes.

Remove bay leaves. Add zucchini, broccoli, spinach, basil, and black pepper. Simmer until broccoli is just tender, about 10 minutes.

Transfer to a blender in several small batches and blend until completely smooth, holding the lid on tightly. Return to pot and heat until steamy. Add salt to taste.

Per 1-cup serving: 107 calories; 6 g protein; 21 g carbohydrate;
0.5 g fat; 4 g fiber; 124-248 mg sodium; calories from protein: 22%;
calories from carbohydrates: 74%; calories from fats: 4%

• • •

Cuban Black Bean Soup
MAKES ABOUT 2 QUARTS SOUP AND 3 CUPS RICE

This flavorful black bean soup is served over marinated rice. A green salad rounds out the meal nicely.

Rice and marinade:
3 cups cooked Brown Rice (page 157)
½ cup finely chopped red onion
1 tablespoon olive oil
3 tablespoons balsamic vinegar

Soup:
1 tablespoon olive oil
1 large onion, chopped

1 large green bell pepper, seeded and diced
6 garlic cloves
1½ teaspoons oregano
1 teaspoon cumin
2 15-ounce cans black beans, undrained
1 tablespoon balsamic vinegar

Prepare the rice: Combine cooked rice with chopped onion, olive oil, and vinegar. Stir to mix. Refrigerate one hour or longer.

For the soup: Heat oil in a large pot; add onion and cook until it begins to soften, about 3 minutes.

Add bell pepper, garlic, oregano, and cumin. Cook, stirring frequently, another 5 minutes.

Add beans with their liquid and 2 cups water. Cover and simmer 30 minutes or longer.

To serve, place about ½ cup of marinated rice in a bowl then cover with a generous ladle of soup.

Per serving (1 cup soup plus ½ cup rice): 250 calories;
9 g protein; 43 g carbohydrate; 5 g fat; 10 g fiber;
414 mg sodium; calories from protein: 15%;
calories from carbohydrates: 68%; calories from fats: 17%

• • •

Creamy Beet Soup

MAKES ABOUT 3 1-CUP SERVINGS

This soup is delicious hot or cold.

1   15-ounce can diced beets
1   cup fortified soy milk or rice milk
2   tablespoons apple juice concentrate
1   teaspoon balsamic vinegar
½ teaspoon dried dill weed

Place diced beets, including liquid, in a blender container. Add milk, apple juice concentrate, vinegar, and dill weed.

Blend on high speed until completely smooth, 2 to 3 minutes. Transfer to a medium saucepan and heat gently until steamy.

Per 1-cup serving: 92 calories; 4 g protein; 17 g carbohydrate; 2 g fat; 4 g fiber; 268 mg sodium; calories from protein: 14%; calories from carbohydrates: 70%; calories from fats: 16%

• • •

Minestrone

MAKES ABOUT 2½ QUARTS (10 1-CUP SERVINGS)

This is a good, basic vegetable soup. You can enhance it with additional vegetables of your choosing. Add fresh-baked bread or muffins and a salad for a satisfying meal.

1   small onion, chopped
4   garlic cloves, minced
1   carrot, cut into chunks
1   celery stalk, sliced, including top
1   potato, scrubbed and cut into chunks
2   tablespoons chopped parsley
2   cups tomato juice
2   cups water or Vegetable Broth (page 180)
1   teaspoon mixed Italian herbs
¼ teaspoon black pepper
1   small zucchini, diced
¼ cup small pasta shells
1   15-ounce can kidney beans, drained
1   cup finely chopped kale, collard greens, or spinach
1   tablespoon chopped fresh basil or 1 teaspoon dried basil

Combine onion, garlic, carrot, celery, potato, and parsley in a large pot. Add tomato juice, water, Italian herbs, and black pepper. Bring to a simmer, then cover and cook 20 minutes.

Add zucchini, pasta, kidney beans, chopped greens, and basil. Cover and simmer until pasta is tender, about 20 minutes. Add extra tomato juice or water for a thinner soup.

Per 1-cup serving: 91 calories; 4 g protein; 19 g carbohydrate;
0.3 g fat; 4 g fiber; 333 mg sodium; calories from protein: 17%;
calories from carbohydrates: 79%; calories from fats: 4%

• • •

Creamy Curried Carrot Soup
MAKES ABOUT 2 QUARTS (8 1-CUP SERVINGS)

This simple soup is a rich source of protective beta-carotene.

1 onion, coarsely chopped
6 carrots, sliced
2 cups Vegetable Broth (page 180)
1 teaspoon curry powder

2 cups fortified soy milk or rice milk
½ to 1 teaspoon salt

Combine onion and carrots in a pot with vegetable broth and curry powder. Cover and simmer until carrots can be easily pierced with a fork,
about 20 minutes.

Transfer 2 to 3 cups of carrots with liquid to a blender; add some of
the milk, and puree until completely smooth, about 2 minutes. Repeat
with remaining carrots.

Return to pot, add more milk if a thinner soup is desired, and heat gently until very hot and steamy.

Per 1-cup serving: 62 calories; 3 g protein; 10 g carbohydrate;
1.5 g fat; 3 g fiber; 290-580 mg sodium; calories from protein: 16%;
calories from carbohydrates: 62%; calories from fats: 22%

• • •

Lima Bean Soup
MAKES ABOUT 1½ QUARTS (6 1-CUP SERVINGS)

*This soup is quick and easy to make. For the best flavor, use fresh basil
and parsley.*

1 onion, chopped
2 garlic cloves, minced
1 cup crushed tomatoes
2 cups shredded cabbage
¼ cup finely chopped fresh basil
1 15-ounce can lima beans,
   drained, or 1½ cups frozen lima
   beans

⅛ teaspoon black pepper
2 cups Vegetable Broth (page
   180), or water
1 cup unsweetened fortified soy
   milk
2 tablespoons chopped fresh
   parsley
½ teaspoon salt

Heat ½ cup water in a large pot; add onion and garlic and cook, stirring occasionally, until soft, about 5 minutes.

Stir in tomatoes, cabbage, basil, lima beans, pepper, and vegetable broth. Cover and simmer 15 minutes.

Transfer about 3 cups of the soup to a blender. Add soy milk and fresh parsley, then blend until smooth, using a low speed and holding the lid on tightly. Return to pot and add salt to taste. Heat gently until hot and steamy.

Per 1-cup serving: 109 calories; 6 g protein; 21 g carbohydrate; 0.7 g fat; 5 g fiber; 416 mg sodium; calories from protein: 20%; calories from carbohydrates: 74%; calories from fats: 6%

• • •

Mexican Corn Chowder

MAKES ABOUT 2½ QUARTS (10 1-CUP SERVINGS)

This soup is spicy and flavorful with no added fat.

2 or 3 cups peeled and diced potato (about 1 pound)
2 cups Vegetable Broth (page 180), or water
1 yellow onion, chopped
2 garlic cloves, minced
1 red bell pepper, diced
1 teaspoon ground cumin
1 teaspoon basil
½ teaspoon salt
¼ teaspoon turmeric
¼ teaspoon black pepper
2 15-ounce cans corn
1 4-ounce can diced green chilies
1 to 2 cups fortified soy milk or rice milk

Place potatoes in a pot with vegetable broth. Cover and simmer until tender, about 20 minutes.

In a separate pan, heat ½ cup water and cook onion, garlic, and bell pepper over medium heat until soft, about 5 minutes. Add cumin, basil, salt, turmeric, and black pepper and cook 5 minutes, stirring often.

When potatoes are tender, mash them in their cooking water and add onion mixture.

Blend one can of corn, with its liquid, until smooth, 2 to 3 minutes, then add it to the soup.

Add remaining can of corn, diced chilies, and 1 cup of milk. Stir to mix. Add more milk if a thinner soup is desired.

Heat gently until very hot and steamy.

Per 1-cup serving: 126 calories; 4 g protein; 27 g carbohydrate; 1 g fat; 3 g fiber; 373 mg sodium; calories from protein: 13%; calories from carbohydrates: 78%; calories from fats: 9%

• • •

Gazpacho

MAKES ABOUT 3 QUARTS (12 1-CUP SERVINGS)

This cool and tangy Spanish soup is perfect for a hot summer day.

2 cucumbers, peeled, seeded, and diced

1 green bell pepper, seeded and diced

3 ripe tomatoes, diced

½ cup finely chopped red onion

3 garlic cloves, pressed

¾ cup roasted red peppers, finely chopped

8 cups vegetable juice (such as V-8) or tomato juice

¾ cup salsa

1 teaspoon finely minced jalapeño pepper, or to taste

Combine all ingredients in a large pot or bowl. Stir to mix, then chill 2 to 3 hours before serving.

Per 1-cup serving: 62 calories; 2 g protein; 13 g carbohydrate; 0.2 g fat; 2 g fiber; 521 mg sodium; calories from protein: 13%; calories from carbohydrates: 83%; calories from fats: 4%

● ● ●

Lentil Soup

MAKES ABOUT 2 QUARTS (8 1-CUP SERVINGS)

This hearty soup takes less than an hour to prepare.

1 cup lentils, rinsed

5 cups Vegetable Broth (page 180) or water

1 onion, chopped

1 celery stalk, diced

1 potato, diced

2 garlic cloves, minced

1 teaspoon ground cumin

1 teaspoon ground coriander

1 cup crushed tomatoes

½ cup chopped fresh cilantro

⅛ teaspoon black pepper

½ teaspoon salt

juice of 1 lemon

Combine lentils, broth, onion, celery, potato, and garlic in a large pot. Cover and simmer 30 minutes.

Toast cumin and coriander in a dry skillet over high heat, stirring constantly, until fragrant, about 30 seconds. Add to lentils along with tomatoes, cilantro, and black pepper. Simmer 15 minutes. Add salt to taste. Stir in lemon juice before serving.

Per 1-cup serving: 122 calories; 9 g protein; 23 g carbohydrate; 0.4 g fat; 5 g fiber; 177 mg sodium; calories from protein: 27%; calories from carbohydrates: 70%; calories from fats: 3%

ENTRÉES

Black Bean Chili

MAKES ABOUT 2 QUARTS (8 1-CUP SERVINGS)

This is a mild chili, delicious with brown rice and a green salad. It can also be used as a burrito filling if it is cooked until it thickens. If you like a hotter chili, add some cayenne or finely chopped jalapeño pepper.

1 tablespoon reduced-sodium soy sauce	1 4-ounce can diced green chilies
2 onions, chopped	1 15-ounce can crushed tomatoes
4 garlic cloves, pressed	2 15-ounce cans black beans, undrained
2 teaspoons oregano	¼ teaspoon salt
½ teaspoon cumin	fresh cilantro, chopped
¼ teaspoon black pepper	

Heat ½ cup water and soy sauce in a large pan until steamy. Add onion and garlic. Cook over medium heat, stirring frequently, until onion is soft, about 5 minutes.

Add oregano, cumin, and black pepper and cook 3 minutes, stirring often. Stir in diced chilies, tomatoes, black beans, and salt. Simmer 20 minutes, or longer for a thicker chili.

Per 1-cup serving: 122 calories; 7 g protein; 23 g carbohydrate;
1 g fat; 8 g fiber; 597 mg sodium; calories from protein: 22%;
calories from carbohydrates: 71%; calories from fats: 7%

● ● ●

Spicy Refried Beans

MAKES ABOUT 5 1-CUP SERVINGS

These beans are flavorful with no added fat. Serve them with rice and a green salad, or as a filling for tacos or burritos.

1½ cups dry pinto beans	1 cup crushed or finely chopped tomatoes
4 garlic cloves, minced or pressed	1 4-ounce can diced green chilies
1½ teaspoons cumin	½ to 1 teaspoon salt
¼ teaspoon cayenne	
1 onion, chopped	

Clean and rinse beans, then soak in about 6 cups of water for 6 to 8 hours. Discard soaking water, rinse beans and place in a large pot with 4 cups of fresh water; add the garlic, cumin, and cayenne. Simmer until tender, about 1 hour.

Heat ½ cup water in a large skillet. Add onion and cook until soft, about 5 minutes. Stir in tomatoes and diced chilies. Cook, uncovered, over medium heat for 10 minutes, stirring occasionally.

A cup at a time, add cooked beans, including some cooking liquid, to tomato mixture. Mash some of the beans as you add them. When all the beans have been added, stir to mix, then cook over low heat, stirring frequently, until thickened. Add salt to taste.

Per 1-cup serving: 110 calories; 6 g protein; 22 g carbohydrate; 0.4 g fat; 6 g fiber; 452 mg sodium; calories from protein: 21%; calories from carbohydrates: 76%; calories from fats: 3%

● ● ●

Cabbage Rolls
MAKES 12 ROLLS

Although this recipe seems lengthy, it isn't difficult to prepare, and everything comes together so deliciously in the end that it's well worth the effort. You could save some time by using a commercially prepared marinara sauce.

head green cabbage

Filling:
1   onion, chopped
1   garlic clove, pressed
2½ cups sliced mushrooms (about ½ pound)
½ teaspoon paprika
⅛ teaspoon black pepper
⅛ teaspoon cayenne
2   cups cooked Brown Rice (see page 157)
¼ cup raisins

¼ cup pine nuts

Sauce:
1   small onion, chopped
1   garlic clove, pressed
1   15-ounce can crushed or ground tomatoes
¼ teaspoon basil
¼ teaspoon oregano
¼ teaspoon fennel seeds
⅛ teaspoon thyme
⅛ teaspoon marjoram
⅛ teaspoon black pepper

Remove core from cabbage, then steam whole head until soft, about 20 minutes. Remove from the pot to cool. When cool enough to handle, peel off 12 large leaves and set aside. Chop enough of the remaining cabbage to make 1 cup. Set aside.

To prepare filling, heat ½ cup water in a large skillet or pot. Add onion and cook until soft, about 5 minutes. Add garlic and mushrooms. Continue cooking, stirring occasionally, until mushrooms are soft, about 5 minutes. Stir in paprika, black pepper, and cayenne. Remove from heat and stir in cooked rice, raisins, pine nuts, and reserved chopped cabbage.

To prepare the sauce, heat ½ cup water in a medium pot. Add onion and garlic and cook over high heat, stirring often, until onion is soft, about 5 minutes. Add tomatoes, basil, oregano, fennel seeds, thyme, marjoram, and black pepper. Cover and simmer over medium heat, stirring occasionally, until flavors are blended, about 25 minutes.

Preheat the oven to 350°F.

To assemble the rolls, divide filling among the 12 leaves. Roll each leaf, starting at the core end and tucking in the edges. Arrange in a 9-by-13-inch baking dish, then spoon sauce evenly over top. Bake 25 minutes.

Per roll: 119 calories; 4 g protein; 24 g carbohydrate; 2 g fat;
4 g fiber; 129 mg sodium; calories from protein: 13%;
calories from carbohydrates: 73%; calories from fats: 14%

• • •

Thai Vegetables
MAKES ABOUT 8 1-CUP SERVINGS

This dish is colorful and mildly spicy. Serve it with flavorful basmati or jasmine rice or with Ginger Noodles (page 160).

2 tablespoons reduced-sodium soy sauce
1 onion, thinly sliced
4 garlic cloves, minced
2 small sweet potatoes or yams, peeled and diced
1 15-ounce can crushed tomatoes
2 teaspoons ground coriander
1 teaspoon ground cumin
½ to 1 teaspoon red pepper flakes
½ teaspoon turmeric

½ teaspoon ginger powder, or 2 teaspoons fresh ginger, minced or grated
1 15-ounce can garbanzo beans, including liquid
1 zucchini, diced
1 red bell pepper, seeded and cut into thin strips
2 teaspoons grated lemon peel
1 tablespoon lemon juice

Heat ½ cup water and soy sauce in a large pot. Add onion and garlic and cook 5 minutes.

Add sweet potatoes, tomatoes, coriander, cumin, pepper flakes, turmeric, ginger, and ½ cup water. Cover and simmer, stirring occasionally, until sweet potatoes are just tender, about 15 minutes.

Add garbanzo beans and their liquid, zucchini, bell pepper, and grated lemon peel. Cover and simmer until zucchini is just tender, about 5 minutes.

Stir in lemon juice before serving.

Per 1-cup serving: 160 calories; 5 g protein; 34 g carbohydrate;
1 g fat; 4 g fiber; 328 mg sodium; calories from protein: 11%;
calories from carbohydrates: 82%; calories from fats: 7%

● ● ●

Kasha with Broccoli and Black Bean Sauce

MAKES ABOUT 8 1-CUP SERVINGS

Kasha (toasted buckwheat groats) is sold in natural food stores and some supermarkets.

1 large bunch broccoli	2 tablespoons lemon juice
4 cups boiling water	2 tablespoons tahini (sesame
2 cups kasha	butter)
½ teaspoon salt	½ teaspoon chili powder
1 15-ounce can black beans,	¼ teaspoon cumin
drained	¼ teaspoon coriander
½ cup roasted red pepper, seeded	¼ cup chopped fresh cilantro

Rinse broccoli and remove stems. Cut or break into bite-sized florets. Peel stem, then slice into ½-inch-thick rounds. Set aside.

Add salt and kasha to boiling water in a saucepan, then cover and simmer until all liquid has been absorbed, about 10 minutes.

Combine black beans, red pepper, lemon juice, tahini, chili powder, cumin, coriander, and cilantro in a food processor or blender and process until very smooth.

Steam broccoli over boiling water until it is bright green and just tender, about 5 minutes. Place a spoonful of kasha on a plate, then top it with steamed broccoli and black bean sauce.

Per 1-cup serving: 120 calories; 6 g protein; 18 g carbohydrate;
4 g fat; 5 g fiber; 148 mg sodium; calories from protein: 18%;
calories from carbohydrates: 56%; calories from fats: 26%

● ● ●

Collard Greens with Portobello Mushrooms
MAKES ABOUT 6 CUPS

This hearty and delicious combination is a complete meal when served over basmati or jasmine rice. These aromatic types of rice can be found in Asian markets and large grocery stores.

6 cups cooked basmati or jasmine
      rice

Mushrooms:
2 large Portobello mushrooms
2 teaspoons toasted sesame oil
2 tablespoons red wine
2 tablespoons reduced-sodium soy
   sauce
1 tablespoon balsamic vinegar
garlic cloves, minced

Garbanzos:
1 small onion, sliced into cres-
   cents
2 teaspoons chopped garlic

2 teaspoons chopped fresh ginger
1 15-ounce can garbanzo beans
¼ cup chopped cilantro (optional)
¼ teaspoon turmeric
¼ teaspoon coriander
¼ teaspoon cinnamon
¼ teaspoon cumin
¼ teaspoon black pepper
¼ teaspoon salt

Greens:
1 bunch collard greens
2 teaspoons olive oil
3 garlic cloves, minced
1 tablespoon reduced-sodium soy
   sauce

Prepare rice as directed on package. While rice is cooking, prepare remaining ingredients.

Cut mushrooms into ¼-inch-thick strips. In a large nonstick skillet combine oil, red wine, soy-sauce, balsamic vinegar, and minced garlic. Heat until steamy, then add mushroom strips. Cover and cook over medium heat, turning frequently, until tender when pierced with a sharp knife, about 5 minutes. Remove from pan and set aside.

Without washing the pan, add ½ cup water and sliced onion. Cook over high heat for 3 minutes, stirring occasionally. Reduce heat to medium-high and add garlic and ginger. Continue cooking, stirring often, until onion is soft, about 3 minutes. Stir in garbanzo beans with their liquid, cilantro (if using), turmeric, coriander, cinnamon, cumin, and black pepper. Cover and cook, stirring occasionally, for 15 minutes. Stir in salt. Remove from pan and set aside.

Wash collards, remove stems and chop leaves into ½-inch-wide strips. You should have 6 to 8 cups. Without washing the pan, add olive oil and garlic. Cook over medium-high heat for 30 seconds, then add chopped collards. Cover and cook, stirring often, until just tender, about 4 minutes. Stir in soy sauce, cooked mushrooms, and garbanzo beans. Serve over cooked rice.

Per serving (1 cup collard mixture over 1 cup rice): 193 calories; 6 g protein; 37 g carbohydrate; 3 g fat; 4 g fiber; 285 mg sodium; calories from protein: 11%; calories from carbohydrates: 75%; calories from fats: 14%

● ● ●

Red Beans and Rice

MAKES ABOUT 6 SERVINGS (1 CUP BEANS AND 1 CUP RICE)

1   cup dry red beans
2   teaspoons olive oil
1   large onion, chopped
3   garlic cloves, minced
1   red bell pepper, seeded and
    diced
2½ cups Vegetable Broth
    (page 180)
2   bay leaves

2   teaspoons oregano
1   teaspoon sage
1   teaspoon thyme
½ teaspoon red pepper flakes
2   tablespoons cider vinegar
½ to 1 teaspoon salt
½ teaspoon liquid smoke (optional)
6   cups cooked Brown Rice
    (page 157)

Rinse beans and soak overnight in 5 to 6 cups of water.

Heat oil in a large pot. Add onion and garlic and cook over high heat, stirring frequently, until onion is soft, about 5 minutes.

Stir in bell pepper, vegetable broth, bay leaves, oregano, sage, thyme, and red pepper flakes. Drain and add soaked beans. Cover and simmer, stirring occasionally, until beans are tender, about 1 hour. Remove bay leaves.

Stir in vinegar, salt, and liquid smoke (if using). Serve over steamed brown rice.

Per serving (1 cup beans and 1 cup rice): 252 calories; 9 g protein; 42 g carbohydrate; 3 g fat; 7 g fiber; 560 mg sodium; calories from protein: 13%; calories from carbohydrates: 75%; calories from fats: 12%

● ● ●

Lasagna
Makes 12 servings

Once again soy works its magic, turning a high-fat favorite into a healthy entree.

2 teaspoons olive oil
1 onion, chopped
1 carrot, grated
3 garlic cloves, pressed or minced
2 cups sliced mushrooms (about ½ pound)
1 15-ounce can crushed or ground tomatoes
1 28-ounce can tomato sauce
1 teaspoon basil
1 teaspoon oregano
½ teaspoon thyme
½ teaspoon fennel seeds
⅛ teaspoon cayenne
1 pound firm tofu
½ cup finely chopped parsley
2 tablespoons reduced-sodium soy sauce
1 10-ounce package frozen chopped spinach, thawed and squeezed dry
12 ounces dry lasagna noodles (about 10 noodles), uncooked

Heat oil in a large pot, then add onion and carrot. Cook over high heat, stirring often until onion is soft, about 5 minutes.

Add garlic and mushrooms and continue cooking until mushrooms are soft, about 5 minutes.

Stir in tomatoes, tomato sauce, basil, oregano, thyme, fennel seeds, and cayenne. Simmer 15 minutes.

Preheat oven to 350°F.

Mash tofu in a mixing bowl, then stir in chopped parsley and soy sauce.

To assemble, spread 1 cup of sauce in a 9-by-13-inch (or larger) baking dish. Cover with a layer of uncooked noodles, half the tofu mixture, and half the spinach.

Spread with half of remaining sauce.

Repeat layers of noodles, tofu, spinach, and sauce. Cover tightly with foil and bake until noodles are tender, about 1 hour. Let stand 10 minutes before serving.

Note: This lasagna may be assembled up to a day in advance and baked just before serving. The noodles will soften while the lasagna stands, so the baking time can be reduced to 30 minutes.

Per serving (¹⁄₁₂ of lasagna): 164 calories;
9 g protein; 27 g carbohydrate; 3 g fat; 4 g fiber;
570 mg sodium; calories from protein: 20%;
calories from carbohydrates: 63%; calories from fats: 17%

● ● ●

Black Bean Pueblo Pie

MAKES 12 SERVINGS

This is like lasagna with a Southwestern twist. It is layered, with black bean chili, corn tortillas, spicy tomato sauce, and tangy garbanzo spread.

Beans:

4 cups cooked black beans (or 2 15-ounce cans, drained)
1 15-ounce can crushed tomatoes
½ cup water
2 teaspoons paprika
2 teaspoons chili powder
2 teaspoons onion powder
1 teaspoon garlic powder

Tomato Sauce:

1 large onion, chopped
1 tablespoon minced garlic (about 4 large cloves)
1 28-ounce can crushed tomatoes

4 teaspoons chili powder
2 teaspoons cumin

Garbanzo spread:

1 15-ounce can garbanzo beans, drained
½ cup water-packed roasted red pepper (about 2 peppers)
2 garlic cloves, peeled
1 tablespoon tahini (sesame butter)
3 tablespoons lemon juice
½ teaspoon cumin
12 corn tortillas, torn in half
1 cup chopped green onions

For the beans: Combine black beans, crushed tomatoes, water, paprika, chili powder, onion powder, and garlic powder in a pot. Bring to a simmer, then cover and cook, stirring frequently, for 25 minutes.

To make sauce, heat ½ cup water in a large pot or skillet. Cook onion and garlic over high heat, stirring often, until soft, about 5 minutes. Add tomatoes, chili powder, and cumin. Cover and simmer over medium heat 5 minutes.

Prepare the garbanzo spread: Combine garbanzo beans, roasted peppers, garlic, tahini, and lemon juice in a food processor or blender. Process until very smooth, about 2 minutes.

Preheat oven to 350°F.

Spread ½ to 1 cup of the tomato sauce in a 9-by-13-inch (or larger) baking dish. Cover with a layer of tortillas, then spread with half of the garbanzo spread, using your fingers to hold tortillas in place. Sprinkle with half of the black beans and green onions. Top with half of the tomato sauce.

Repeat layers, ending with tomato sauce. Bake for 25 minutes.

Per serving (1/12 of casserole): 177 calories; 8 g protein; 32 g carbohydrate; 2.5 g fat; 5 g fiber; 172 mg sodium; calories from protein: 17%; calories from carbohydrates: 70%; calories from fats: 13%

• • •

Eggplant Manicotti
MAKES ABOUT 12 MANICOTTI

In this recipe, eggplant is used in place of pasta to wrap up a creamy spinach filling. Serve it with Garlic Bread (page 207) and Mixed Greens with Apples and Walnuts (page 170).

1 large eggplant	½ teaspoon onion powder
olive oil spray	½ teaspoon garlic powder
1 medium onion, chopped	¼ teaspoon grated nutmeg
2 10-ounce packages frozen chopped spinach, thawed	¼ teaspoon salt
	¼ cup whole wheat flour
2 teaspoons basil	2 cups Marinara Sauce (recipe
½ teaspoon oregano	follows)

Preheat broiler. Slice eggplant lengthwise into ¼-inch thick slices (you should have about 12 slices).

Spray a baking sheet with olive oil. Arrange eggplant slices in a single layer, then lightly spray or brush with olive oil. Broil until lightly browned, then turn and cook second side until lightly browned and tender when pierced with a fork. Set aside.

Heat ½ cup water in a large nonstick skillet. Cook onion over high heat, stirring often until dry. Add 2 tablespoons water, stir to loosen any stuck bits of onion, then continue cooking until all the liquid evaporates again.

Repeat this process twice more, then add spinach, basil, oregano, onion powder, garlic powder, nutmeg, and salt. Cook until spinach is very hot, about 4 minutes, then stir in flour. Cook 2 to 3 minutes longer. Set aside to cool.

Preheat oven to 350°F.

Place a spoonful of spinach mixture across the center of each slice of eggplant. Beginning with the narrow end, roll eggplant slice around filling. Arrange in a baking dish, seam side down. Top with about 2 cups of your favorite marinara sauce, or use the recipe that follows.

Cover and bake 20 minutes.

Marinara Sauce:

½ cup water or wine	1 tablespoon apple juice concen-
½ onion, chopped	trate
2 garlic cloves, minced or pressed	1½ teaspoons Italian seasoning
1 15-ounce can chopped or crushed tomatoes	⅛ teaspoon black pepper

Heat water or wine in a large pot. Add onion and garlic and cook over high heat, stirring often, until onion is soft, about 5 minutes.

Add tomatoes, apple juice concentrate, Italian seasoning, and black pepper. Cover and simmer, stirring occasionally, 15 to 20 minutes.

Per manicotti: 72 calories; 3.5 g protein; 16 g carbohydrate;
0.5 g fat; 5 g fiber; 147 mg sodium; calories from protein: 16%;
calories from carbohydrates: 78%; calories from fats: 6%

● ● ●

Stuffed Winter Squash

MAKES 6 SERVINGS

Golden squash halves, mounded with stuffing and topped with apricot sauce make a visual feast worthy of any holiday meal. Use any of the smaller varieties of winter squash, including acorn squash, delicata, sweet dumpling, or kabocha.

3 medium-size winter squash	½ cup dried apricots, chopped
1 tablespoon plus 2 tablespoons reduced-sodium soy sauce, divided	½ teaspoon sage
	½ teaspoon marjoram
	½ teaspoon thyme
1 medium onion, chopped	¼ teaspoon black pepper
2 garlic cloves, minced	2 cups apricot nectar
2 cups sliced mushrooms (about ½ pound)	¼ teaspoon ground ginger
	¼ teaspoon ground coriander
1 cup sliced celery (2 large ribs)	¼ teaspoon cinnamon
¼ cup finely chopped parsley	2 tablespoons maple syrup
4 cups cubed whole wheat bread	2 teaspoons cornstarch

Cut squash in half and scoop out seeds. Steam until tender when pierced with a fork, about 20 to 30 minutes.

Heat ½ cup water and 1 tablespoon of the soy sauce in a large pot. Add onion, garlic, mushrooms, and celery. Cover and cook over medium heat, stirring occasionally, until onion is soft, about 5 minutes. Remove from heat.

Stir in parsley, bread cubes, dried apricots, sage, marjoram, thyme, and black pepper. The mixture should be moist enough to hold together, but not wet. If it is too dry, add a small amount of water or vegetable stock.

Preheat oven to 350°F. Divide stuffing mixture evenly among squash halves and bake 20 minutes.

Meanwhile, mix apricot nectar with ginger, coriander, cinnamon, maple syrup, cornstarch, and the remaining 2 tablespoons of soy sauce.

Bring to a simmer, stirring constantly, and cook until clear and slightly thickened, about 2 minutes. Remove from heat.

Make a depression in the top of the stuffing on each squash. Fill with apricot sauce. Serve remaining sauce on the side.

Per ½ squash: 312 calories; 8 g protein; 75 g carbohydrate; 2 g fat;
14 g fiber; 410 mg sodium; calories from protein: 9%;
calories from carbohydrates: 87%; calories from fats: 4%

• • •

Barbecue-style Portobellos
MAKES 2 SERVINGS

Large meaty portobello mushrooms make a delicious meal when they're simmered in a spicy sauce and served with Polenta (page 159), Brown Rice (page 157), pasta, or French bread.

2 large Portobello mushrooms
½ cup vegetable juice (Low-Sodium V-8, Very Veggie, or similar)
¼ cup apple juice concentrate
½ cup roasted red peppers
1 tablespoon reduced-sodium soy sauce
1 tablespoon seasoned rice vinegar
2 teaspoons chili powder
½ teaspoon garlic powder
¼ teaspoon black pepper

Clean mushrooms and remove stems. Cut into ½-inch wide strips.

Combine vegetable juice, apple juice, roasted red peppers, soy sauce, vinegar, chili powder, and garlic powder in a blender. Process until smooth, and then transfer mixture to a nonstick skillet and heat until bubbly.

Add mushroom strips, turning to coat evenly with sauce. Cover and cook over medium-high heat, turning occasionally, until mushrooms are tender, about 10 minutes. Serve immediately.

Per ½ of recipe: 70 calories; 3 g protein; 14.5 g carbohydrate;
0.4 g fat; 2 g fiber; 453 mg sodium; calories from protein: 19%;
calories from carbohydrates: 76%; calories from fats: 5%

VEGETABLES

Broccoli with Fat-Free Dressing
MAKES 4 TO 6 SERVINGS

Seasoned rice vinegar makes a sweet-sour dressing that is a perfect addition to lightly steamed broccoli. Try it on steamed green beans, too.

1 large bunch broccoli	1 teaspoon stone-ground mustard
¼ cup seasoned rice vinegar	1 garlic clove, pressed or minced

Break broccoli into bite-size flowerets; you should have about 4 cups. Peel stems and slice into ¼-inch thick rounds. Steam until just tender, about 5 minutes.

While broccoli is steaming, combine vinegar, mustard, and garlic in a serving bowl. Add steamed broccoli and toss to mix. Serve immediately.

Variation: For a tasty salad, plunge the steamed broccoli into ice water until it is completely chilled; drain, then toss with the dressing.

Per ½-cup serving: 20 calories; 1 g protein; 4 g carbohydrate; 0.2 g fat; 1 g fiber; 160 mg sodium; calories from protein: 24%; calories from carbohydrates: 68%; calories from fats: 8%

● ● ●

Braised Collards or Kale
MAKES 3 1-CUP SERVINGS

Collard greens and kale are rich sources of calcium and beta-carotene as well as other minerals and vitamins. One of the tastiest—and easiest—ways to prepare them is with a bit of soy sauce and plenty of garlic. Try to purchase young tender greens, as these have the best flavor and texture.

1 bunch collard greens or kale (6 to 8 cups chopped)	1 teaspoon balsamic vinegar
1 teaspoon olive oil	2 to 3 garlic cloves, minced
2 teaspoons reduced-sodium soy sauce	

Wash greens, remove stems, then cut leaves into ½-inch wide strips.

Combine olive oil, soy sauce, vinegar, garlic, and ¼ cup water in a large pot or skillet. Cook over high heat about 30 seconds. Reduce heat to medium-high, add chopped greens, and toss to mix. Cover and cook, stirring often, until greens are tender, about 5 minutes.

Per 1-cup serving: 106 calories; 6 g protein; 18 g carbohydrate; 2 g fat; 6 g fiber; 132 mg sodium; calories from protein: 20%; calories from carbohydrates: 60%; calories from fats: 20%

● ● ●

Bok Choy

MAKES 3 1-CUP SERVINGS

Bok choy is another calcium-rich dark leafy green. The stems are crisp and tender, and can be sliced and cooked with the leaves.

2 bunches bok choy (about 6 cups chopped)
1 teaspoon olive oil
2 teaspoons reduced-sodium soy sauce

2 to 3 garlic cloves, minced
1 teaspoon balsamic vinegar

Wash bok choy, then slice leaves and stems into ½-inch strips.

Combine olive oil, soy sauce, garlic and ¼ cup water in a large pot or skillet. Cook over high heat about 30 seconds, then add bok choy and toss to mix.

Reduce heat to medium-high, then cover and cook, stirring often, until tender, about 5 minutes. Sprinkle with balsamic vinegar and toss to mix.

> Per 1-cup serving: 60 calories; 4 g protein; 8 g carbohydrate;
> 2 g fat; 2 g fiber; 306 mg sodium; calories from protein: 23%;
> calories from carbohydrates: 41%; calories from fats: 36%

● ● ●

Winter Vegetable Medley

MAKES 3 1-CUP SERVINGS

This nutritious combination of broccoli, cauliflower, and carrots is color-ful and delicious.

1 cup broccoli florets
1 cup cauliflower florets
1 cup carrots, cut on the diagonal into thin slices

1 tablespoon lemon juice
1 tablespoon Sesame Salt (page 174)

Steam vegetables over boiling water until just tender, about 5 minutes. Sprinkle with lemon juice and sesame salt.

> Per 1-cup serving: 58 calories; 2 g protein; 10 g carbohydrate;
> 2 g fat; 4 g fiber; 96 mg sodium; calories from protein: 16%;
> calories from carbohydrates: 60%; calories from fats: 24%

● ● ●

Beets in Dill Sauce

MAKES ABOUT 8 ½-CUP SERVINGS

These sweet and sour beets are delicious hot or cold. Serve them as a side dish or add them to a green salad.

4   medium beets (about 4 cups sliced)
2   tablespoons lemon juice
1   tablespoon stone-ground mustard
1   tablespoon cider vinegar
1   tablespoon apple juice concentrate
1   teaspoon dried dill weed or 1 tablespoon fresh dill, chopped

Wash and peel beets, then slice into ¼-inch-thick rounds. Steam over boiling water until tender when pierced with a fork, about 20 minutes.

Mix lemon juice, mustard, vinegar, apple juice concentrate, and dill in a serving bowl. Add beets and toss to mix. Serve immediately, or chill before serving.

Per ½-cup serving: 44 calories; 2 g protein; 10 g carbohydrate; 0.3 g fat; 1.5 g fiber; 113 mg sodium; calories from protein: 14%; calories from carbohydrates: 81%; calories from fats: 5%

● ● ●

Delicata Squash

MAKES 6 SERVINGS

The cylindrical, green-and-yellow-striped delicata squash has sweet yellow flesh. Look for it in stores from September to November.

3   delicata squash
1   tablespoon Sesame Salt (page 174)
freshly ground black pepper

Cut squash in half length-wise and remove seeds. Steam over boiling water until tender when pierced with a fork, about 15 minutes.

Sprinkle with Sesame Salt and pepper. Serve immediately.

Per ½ squash: 56 calories; 3 g protein; 11 g carbohydrate; 1 g fat; 3 g fiber; 30 mg sodium; calories from protein: 17%; calories from carbohydrates: 65%; calories from fats: 18%

● ● ●

Carrots in Orange Sauce

MAKES ABOUT 6 ½-CUP SERVINGS

The radiant golden color of these carrots tells you they're loaded with protective beta-carotene.

4 or 5 medium carrots	1 teaspoon reduced-sodium soy
¾ cup orange juice	sauce
1½ teaspoons cornstarch	¼ teaspoon dill weed
1 tablespoon apple juice concentrate	

Scrub carrots and cut into ¼-inch-thick slices. You should have 2 to 3 cups. Steam until just tender when pierced with a fork.

Combine orange juice, cornstarch, apple juice concentrate, soy sauce, and dill weed in a saucepan. Whisk smooth, then bring to a simmer over medium heat, stirring constantly. Cook until sauce is clear and slightly thickened.

Add carrots to sauce and heat through. Serve hot or cold.

Per ½-cup serving: 27 calories; 0.4 g protein; 6 g carbohydrate; 1 g fat; 0.4 g fiber; 33 mg sodium; calories from protein: 6%; calories from carbohydrates: 91%; calories from fats: 3%

● ● ●

Braised Cabbage

MAKES ABOUT 3 ½-CUP SERVINGS

The mellow, sweet flavor of braised cabbage goes well with any meal.

2 cups green cabbage, coarsely chopped	salt
½ teaspoon caraway seeds (optional)	black pepper

Heat ½ cup water in a skillet or saucepan. Stir in cabbage and caraway seeds, if using. Cover and cook over medium heat until cabbage is just tender, about 4 minutes. Sprinkle with salt and pepper to taste.

Per ½-cup serving: 12 calories; 1 g protein; 3 g carbohydrate; 0.1 g fat; 1 g fiber; 56 mg sodium; calories from protein: 20%; calories from carbohydrates: 72%; calories from fats: 8%

● ● ●

Cooking Potatoes, Sweet Potatoes, Yams, and Winter Squash

Potatoes, sweet potatoes, and winter squash are traditionally baked, but steaming and microwaving are also excellent methods for cooking these nutritious vegetables. In addition to being quick and easy, the vegetables stay moist and flavorful.

Steaming

To steam potatoes, yams, or sweet potatoes, simply scrub them (or peel them if you prefer) and arrange them on a steamer rack. Cook in a covered pot over simmering water until tender when pierced with a fork. This will take between 15 and 40 minutes, depending on their size. For quicker cooking, cut them into cubes or slices before steaming.

To steam winter squash, cut it in half and scoop out the seeds with a spoon. Cut it into wedges or other conveniently sized pieces and arrange on a steamer rack. Place in a pot, then cover and cook over medium heat until the squash is tender when pierced with a fork, between 15 and 30 minutes, depending on the size and freshness of the squash.

Microwave cooking

Russet Potatoes

2 medium potatoes

Pierce potato in several places with a fork. Place in microwave on rotating surface or turn midway during cooking. Microwave 7 to 8 minutes on high. Pierce with a fork to test for doneness. Crisp potato skins by placing in a toaster oven for a short time.

Sweet Potatoes or Yams

2 medium yams

Place yams in shallow covered casserole. Do not add water. Microwave 6 minutes on high, then turn yams over and microwave another 4 minutes. Test for doneness with a fork.

Butternut or Acorn Squash

1 squash

Cut squash in half and remove seeds. Place cut side down in a shallow dish. Do not add water. Microwave on high for 8 minutes. Turn squash right side up and cook another 6 minutes on high.

Summer Succotash

MAKES ABOUT 8 1-CUP SERVINGS

This colorful vegetable dish goes well with baked sweet potatoes and Brown Rice (page 157).

2 teaspoons olive oil
1 large onion, chopped
2 garlic cloves, minced
1½ teaspoons dried basil
¼ teaspoon black pepper
1 large yellow zucchini, cut into ½-inch cubes (about 2 cups)
2 cups (packed) finely chopped fresh kale

1 9-ounce package frozen green beans
1 15-ounce can corn, including liquid
2 tablespoons reduced-sodium soy sauce

Heat oil in a large nonstick skillet and cook onions and garlic until soft, about 5 minutes.

Rub basil between your hands to crush it. Add to onions along with black pepper, zucchini, and chopped kale. Stir to mix, then cook 2 minutes.

Add corn with its liquid. Cover and cook over medium heat, stirring occasionally, until kale and zucchini are tender, about 5 minutes. Stir in soy sauce before serving.

Per 1-cup serving: 69 calories; 3 g protein; 13 g carbohydrate;
2 g fat; 2 g fiber; 274 mg sodium; calories from protein: 14%;
calories from carbohydrates: 68%; calories from fats: 18%

• • •

Mashed Potatoes and Kale

MAKES ABOUT 6 1-CUP SERVINGS

4 medium russet potatoes
1 cup unsweetened fortified soy milk
1 teaspoon salt
⅛ teaspoon black pepper

1 bunch kale
1 tablespoon reduced-sodium soy sauce
2 or 3 cloves garlic, minced

Scrub potatoes, peel if desired, and cut into chunks. Place in a large pot with 1 cup of water. Cover and cook over medium heat until tender when pierced with a fork, about 20 minutes.

Without draining, mash potatoes, then add soy milk, salt, and pepper.

Wash kale, remove stems, and finely chop leaves (you should have about 3 cups).

Heat ½ cup water in a large pot or skillet. Add soy sauce and garlic and cook 30 seconds. Stir in chopped kale, then cover and cook over medium heat until tender, about 5 minutes.

When kale is tender, mix it with the mashed potatoes.

Per 1-cup serving: 186 calories; 6 g protein; 40 g carbohydrate; 0.6 g fat; 4 g fiber; 470 mg sodium; calories from protein: 12%; calories from carbohydrates: 85%; calories from fats: 3%

● ● ●

Curried Potatoes

MAKES ABOUT 5 1-CUP SERVINGS

Serve these colorful, spicy potatoes with chutney and a lentil or bean soup.

4 large red potatoes
2 teaspoons whole mustard seed
½ teaspoon turmeric
½ teaspoon ground cumin
¼ teaspoon ground ginger

⅛ teaspoon cayenne
⅛ teaspoon black pepper
1 onion, chopped
1½ tablespoons soy sauce

Scrub potatoes, then cut into ¼-inch cubes. Steam until tender when pierced with a fork, 10 to 15 minutes. Cool completely.

Toast mustard seed, turmeric, cumin, ginger, cayenne, and black pepper in a large, dry nonstick skillet for 1 to 2 minutes, stirring constantly. Carefully pour in ½ cup water (there will be some splattering).

Add chopped onion and cook, stirring frequently, until soft, about 5 minutes.

Add cooled potatoes, ½ cup water, and soy sauce. Cover and cook over medium heat for 5 minutes. Stir before serving.

Per 1-cup serving: 182 calories; 4 g protein; 42 g carbohydrate;
0.2 g fat; 4 g fiber; 202 mg sodium; calories from protein: 9%;
calories from carbohydrates: 90%; calories from fats: 1%

• • •

Mashed Potatoes
MAKES ABOUT 10 ½-CUP SERVINGS

Serve with Brown Gravy (page 173) and enjoy this traditional favorite to your heart's content!

4   russet potatoes, peeled and diced
1   cup unsweetened fortified soy
    milk or rice milk
¼ teaspoon onion powder
¼ teaspoon garlic powder
½ teaspoon salt

1½ tablespoons rice flour
2   tablespoons potato flour
½ cup Corn Butter (page 172), or
    1 tablespoon non-hydrogenated
    margarine

Put potatoes and 2 cups water in a saucepan. Simmer until potatoes are tender when pierced with a fork, about 10 minutes. Drain, reserving liquid. Mash potatoes.

Pour milk, onion powder, garlic powder, salt, rice flour, potato flour, and Corn Butter or margarine into a blender. Blend until completely smooth, about 1 minute. Add to mashed potatoes and stir to mix.

Per ½-cup serving: 85 calories;
2 g protein; 18 g carbohydrate; 1 g fat; 2 g fiber;
140 mg sodium; calories from protein: 11%;
calories from carbohydrates: 81%; calories from fats: 8%

• • •

Sweet Potatoes with Pineapple
MAKES 4 1-CUP SERVINGS

Golden and delicious, these are very easy to prepare.

2   medium sweet potatoes or yams,
    unpeeled

1   cup crushed pineapple in juice

Scrub sweet potatoes or yams and steam over boiling water until tender, about 25 minutes. Remove from steamer and cool slightly.

When cool enough to handle, cut a lengthwise slit and squeeze ends to open. Leaving the flesh in the skin, mash it slightly with a fork.

Mix in 2 to 3 tablespoons of undrained crushed pineapple, then fill cavities with remaining pineapple.

Variation: Peel cooked yams when they are cool enough to handle. Mash flesh and mix in pineapple, including liquid.

Per 1-cup serving: 192 calories; 2 g protein; 46 g carbohydrate;
0.4 g fat; 4 g fiber; 20 mg sodium; calories from protein: 6%;
calories from carbohydrates: 92%; calories from fats: 2%

• • •

Edamame (Whole Green Soybeans)
MAKES ABOUT 3 CUPS (6 ½-CUP SERVINGS)

Add some soy to your life with edamame. This traditional Japanese appetizer is served in the pod, like peanuts in the shell. Simply pop the soybeans out of the pod and enjoy!

1   pound green soybeans   ½ teaspoon salt (optional)
    (edamame)

Bring 6 cups of water to a boil in a large pot. Add soybeans and return to a boil. Cook 10 minutes. Drain well and toss with salt. Shell beans before eating.

Per ½ cup serving: 107 calories; 9 g protein; 8 g carbohydrate; 5 g fat;
3 g fiber; 11–99 mg sodium; calories from protein: 33%;
calories from carbohydrates: 29%; calories from fats: 38%

• • •

French Green Lentils
MAKES ABOUT 6 1-CUP SERVINGS

French green lentils have a distinctive and delicious peppery flavor. Look for them in natural food stores and specialty food markets. If brown lentils may be used as a substitute, increase the cooking time to 50 minutes.

1 cup French green lentils	1 teaspoon cumin
4 cups Vegetable Broth (page 180)	1 teaspoon coriander
1 large onion, chopped	½ teaspoon powdered ginger
½ cup cilantro, chopped	⅛ to ¼ teaspoon cayenne
1 teaspoon black mustard seeds	½ teaspoon salt
1 teaspoon turmeric	

Rinse lentils and place in a large pot with vegetable broth, onion, and cilantro.

Combine mustard seeds, turmeric, cumin, coriander, ginger, and cayenne in a small skillet. Toast over medium-high heat, stirring constantly, until spices are fragrant and just begin to smoke, about 2 minutes. Add to lentils.

Cover and simmer until lentils are tender, about 30 minutes. Add salt to taste.

Per 1-cup serving: 124 calories; 9 g protein; 22 g carbohydrate;
0.3 g fat; 5 g fiber; 182 mg sodium; calories from protein: 29%;
calories from carbohydrates: 68%; calories from fats: 3%

● ● ●

Roasted Red Peppers

Roasted red peppers are delicious additions to salads, sauces, and soups. You can purchase water-packed roasted peppers in most grocery stores, or you can roast your own as described below.

1 (or more) large, firm red bell peppers

Wash pepper and place it over an open flame (such as a gas burner on the stove) or under the oven broiler. Turn pepper with tongs until skin is evenly charred on all sides.

Transfer to a bowl and cover with a plate. Let stand 15 minutes, then rub off charred skin. Cut pepper in half, saving any juice, and remove seeds. Use immediately or refrigerate or freeze for later use.

Per pepper: 20 calories; 0.6 g protein; 5 g carbohydrate;
0.1 g fat; 1 g fiber; 1 mg sodium; calories from protein: 11%;
calories from carbohydrates: 83%; calories from fats: 6%

● ● ●

Roasted Garlic

Roasted garlic is a delicious appetizer or accompaniment to a meal. Serve it spread onto crusty French bread or mash it and add it to salad dressings. Store in a sealed container in the refrigerator for up to 2 weeks.

1 or more whole garlic heads

Preheat oven or toaster oven to 375°F.

Select heads of garlic with large cloves. Place entire bulb in a small baking dish and bake until cloves feel soft when pressed, about 35 minutes.

Microwave variation: Place 1 large head of garlic in microwave. Cook on high for 2 minutes, 10 seconds. Test for doneness with a fork.

Per bulb: 45 calories; 2 g protein; 10 g carbohydrate;
0.1 g fat; 0.6 g fiber; 5 mg sodium; calories from protein: 16%;
calories from carbohydrates: 81%; calories from fats: 3%

BREADS AND DESSERTS

Garlic Bread
MAKES ABOUT 20 SLICES

Roasted garlic makes a delicious, fat-free garlic bread. Choose heads with nice big cloves for easy peeling.

2   Roasted Garlic heads (see previous recipe)
1 to 2 teaspoons mixed Italian herbs
½ teaspoon salt
1   baguette or loaf of French bread, sliced

Preheat oven to 350°F.
Peel roasted cloves, or squeeze flesh from skin, and place in a bowl.
Mash with a fork, then mix in Italian herbs and salt.
Spread on sliced bread. Wrap tightly in foil and bake for 20 minutes.

Per slice: 88 calories; 3 g protein; 17 g carbohydrate;
1 g fat; 1 g fiber; 229 mg sodium; calories from protein: 13%;
calories from carbohydrates: 76%; calories from fats: 11%

● ● ●

Quick and Easy Brown Bread
MAKES 1 LOAF (ABOUT 20 SLICES)

This bread is made with healthful whole wheat and contains no added fat or oil. Serve it plain or with Pineapple Apricot Sauce (page 179).

1½ cups fortified soy milk or rice milk
2   tablespoons vinegar
3   cups whole wheat pastry flour
2   teaspoons baking soda
½ teaspoon salt
½ cup molasses
½ cup raisins

Preheat oven to 325°F.

Mix milk with vinegar and set aside.

In a large bowl, combine flour, baking soda, and salt. Stir to mix.

Add milk mixture and molasses. Stir to mix, then stir in raisins. Do not overmix.

Spread evenly in 5-by-9 inch nonstick or oil-sprayed loaf pan (pan should be about half full). Bake one hour.

Per slice: 100 calories; 3 g protein; 22 g carbohydrate;
1 g fat; 2 g fiber; 186 mg sodium; calories from protein: 12%;
calories from carbohydrates: 82%; calories from fats: 6%

• • •

Blueberry Muffins

MAKES 12 MUFFINS

These delicious muffins are loaded with protective blueberries.

vegetable oil cooking spray
1½ cups unbleached flour
1½ cups barley flour
¼ cup sugar or other sweetener
2 teaspoons baking soda
½ teaspoon salt
1½ cups fortified soy milk or rice milk

⅓ cup orange juice concentrate
2 tablespoons seasoned rice vinegar
2 tablespoons canola oil
2 cups blueberries, fresh or frozen

Preheat oven to 350°F. Spray a 12-cup muffin tin with cooking spray.

Mix flours, sugar, baking soda, and salt.

In a large bowl combine milk, orange juice concentrate, vinegar, and oil. Add flour mixture and stir just to mix. Stir in blueberries.

Spoon batter into prepared muffin cups, filling to just below tops.

Bake until lightly browned and tops of muffins bounce back when pressed, about 25 to 30 minutes. Remove from oven and let stand about 5 minutes, then remove from pan and cool on a rack.

Per muffin: 229 calories; 6 g protein; 45 g carbohydrate;
3 g fat; 5 g fiber; 306 mg sodium; calories from protein: 10%;
calories from carbohydrates: 77%; calories from fats: 13%

• • •

Berry Cobbler
MAKES 9 SERVINGS

This cobbler is a simple and delicious way to enjoy healthful berries!

Berry mixture:
5 to 6 cups fresh or frozen berries
(blueberries, blackberries,
raspberries, or a mixture of
these)
¼ cup whole wheat pastry flour
½ cup sugar

Topping:
1 cup whole wheat pastry flour
2 tablespoons sugar
1½ teaspoons baking powder
¼ teaspoon salt
⅔ cup fortified soy milk or rice
milk

Preheat oven to 375°F.

Spread berries in a 9-by-9-inch baking dish. Mix in flour and sugar. Place in oven until hot, about 15 minutes.

Meanwhile, prepare topping: Mix flour, sugar, baking powder, and salt in a bowl. Add milk and stir until batter is smooth.

Spread evenly over hot berries (don't worry if they're not completely covered), then bake until golden brown, 25 to 30 minutes.

Per serving (⅑ of cobbler): 164 calories;
3 g protein; 38 g carbohydrate; 1 g fat; 6 g fiber;
123 mg sodium; calories from protein: 8%;
calories from carbohydrates: 87%; calories from fats: 5%

● ● ●

Fresh Peach Crisp
MAKES 9 SERVINGS

What a perfect way to enjoy summer's juicy golden peaches! At other times of year you can use frozen peach slices.

Peaches:
5 to 6 medium-size fresh peaches
1 tablespoon cornstarch
1 tablespoon maple syrup
1 tablespoon lemon juice

Topping:
1¼ cups Grape-Nuts cereal

1½ cups rolled oats
½ cup Corn Butter (see recipe page
172)
½ cup maple syrup
½ teaspoon cinnamon
1 teaspoon vanilla

Preheat oven to 350°F.

Peel and slice peaches (you should have about 6 cups). Toss with cornstarch, maple syrup, and lemon juice. Spread evenly in a 9-by-9-inch baking dish.

Mix Grape-Nuts, rolled oats, Corn Butter, maple syrup, cinnamon, and vanilla. Spread over peaches. Bake 25 minutes.

Per serving (⅑ of crisp): 189 calories; 4 g protein; 42 g carbohydrate; 1g
fat; 4 g fiber; 138 mg sodium; calories from protein: 9%;
calories from carbohydrates: 85%; calories from fats: 6%

● ● ●

Prune Whip
MAKES 3 SERVINGS

Carob powder, which is naturally sweet, adds delicious flavor to this simple pudding. Look for carob powder in your natural food store.

1 cup pitted prunes   2 tablespoons maple syrup
2 tablespoons carob powder

Place prunes and 1 cup water in a saucepan. Cover and simmer until prunes are soft.

Transfer to a food processor or blender. Add carob powder and maple syrup and puree. Serve warm or chilled.

Per ½-cup serving: 127 calories; 1 g protein; 33 g carbohydrate;
0.2 g fat; 6 g fiber; 4 mg sodium; calories from protein: 3%;
calories from carbohydrates: 96%; calories from fats: 1%

● ● ●

Brown Rice Pudding
MAKES 6 ½-CUP SERVINGS

This stovetop pudding is also great for breakfast.

1½ cups fortified vanilla soy milk   ¼ cup maple syrup
1 tablespoon cornstarch   ⅓ cup raisins
2 cups cooked Brown Rice (page   ¼ teaspoon cinnamon
   157)   1 teaspoon vanilla

Whisk milk and cornstarch together in a medium saucepan. Add cooked rice, maple syrup, raisins, and cinnamon.

Simmer over medium heat 3 minutes, stirring constantly. Remove from heat and stir in vanilla. Serve warm or cold.

Per ½-cup serving: 155 calories; 3 g protein; 32 g carbohydrate;
2 g fat; 2 g fiber; 99 mg sodium; calories from protein: 9%;
calories from carbohydrates: 81%; calories from fats: 10%

● ● ●

Dried Fruit Compote
MAKES ABOUT 8 ½-CUP SERVINGS

Serve this delicious compote for breakfast on hot cereal or for dessert with Brown Rice Pudding (page 212).

½ cup raisins
½ cup pitted prunes
½ cup dried figs, halved

½ cup dried peaches or apricots
½ cup white grape juice concentrate or apple juice concentrate

Combine raisins, prunes, figs, peaches, and white grape juice concentrate in a saucepan. Add just enough water to cover fruit.

Cover and simmer 15 minutes. Serve warm or cold.

Per ½-cup serving: 116 calories; 1 g protein; 30 g carbohydrate; 0.3 g fat; 2 g fiber; 3 mg sodium; calories from protein: 4%; calories from carbohydrates: 94%; calories from fats: 2%

● ● ●

Fruit Gel
MAKES 8 ½-CUP SERVINGS

This is an all natural alternative to Jell-O! Agar powder and kudzu ("kood-zoo") are natural plant-based thickeners available in natural food stores.

1½ cups strawberries, fresh or frozen
¾ cups apple juice concentrate

½ teaspoon agar powder
1 tablespoon kudzu powder
2 cups blueberries, fresh or frozen

Chop strawberries by hand or in a food processor.

Place in a pan with apple juice concentrate, ½ cup water, agar, and kudzu powder. Stir to mix.

Bring to a simmer and cook 3 minutes, stirring often. Remove from heat and chill completely.

Fold in blueberries and transfer to serving dishes.

Variations: Two cups of fresh or frozen blackberries or raspberries, or chopped peaches or mango may be substituted for the blueberries.

Per ½-cup serving: 77 calories; 0.5 g protein; 19 g carbohydrate; 0.2 g fat; 2 g fiber; 9 mg sodium; calories from protein: 2%; calories from carbohydrates: 95%; calories from fats: 3%

● ● ●

Blueberry Pudding

MAKES 5 ½-CUP SERVINGS

Enjoy blueberries in this quick and easy pudding.

1   12.3-ounce package Mori-Nu
     Lite silken tofu (firm or extra
     firm)
1   cup blueberries, fresh or frozen

2   tablespoons lemon juice
⅓   cup sugar or other sweetener
¼   teaspoon salt

Place all ingredients in a food processor or blender and blend until completely smooth. Spoon into serving bowls and chill.

Per ½-cup serving: 93 calories; 4 g protein; 19 g carbohydrate;
1 g fat; 1 g fiber; 150 mg sodium; calories from protein: 17%;
calories from carbohydrates: 75%; calories from fats: 8%

• • •

Holiday Fruitcake

MAKES 2 LOAVES (40 SLICES)

This delicious holiday bread can be easily modified by using different combinations of dried fruit.

vegetable cooking oil spray
1½ cups soy milk or rice milk
2   tablespoons vinegar
3   cups whole wheat pastry flour
2   teaspoons baking soda
½   teaspoon salt
¼   cup molasses

¼ cup maple syrup or rice syrup
1   cup dark raisins
1   cup chopped dried figs
1   cup golden raisins
½   cup chopped pitted dates
½   cup chopped dried apricots

Preheat oven to 325°F.

Coat inside of two 5-by-9 inch loaf pans with cooking spray. Mix milk and vinegar and set aside.

In a large bowl mix flour, soda, and salt. Add milk-vinegar mixture, molasses, and maple syrup. Mix well, then stir in dried fruit.

Divide batter between the two prepared loaf pans and bake one hour.

Per slice: 90 calories; 2 g protein; 22 g carbohydrate; 0.4 g fat;
2 g fiber; 94 mg sodium; calories from protein: 8%;
calories from carbohydrates: 88%; calories from fats: 4%

• • •

Blueberry Freeze
MAKES 3 TO 4 1-CUP SERVINGS

By varying the amount of soy milk or rice milk, you can make this frozen dessert thick enough to eat with a spoon or thin enough to drink through a straw. Either style is a delicious way to enjoy the benefits of blueberries. To freeze bananas, peel them, then cut or break into 1-inch pieces. Pack loosely into airtight containers or freezer bags.

1 cup frozen blueberries
1 cup frozen banana chunks

1½ to 3 cups fortified vanilla soy milk or rice milk
¼ cup apple juice concentrate

Place all ingredients in a blender. Process on high speed until smooth, 2 to 3 minutes, stopping blender occasionally to move unblended fruit to the center with a spatula. Serve immediately.

Per 1-cup serving: 111 calories; 2 g protein; 25 g carbohydrate; 1 g fat; 2 g fiber; 18 mg sodium; calories from protein: 7%; calories from carbohydrates: 85%; calories from fats: 8%

BEVERAGES

Apricot Smoothie
MAKES ABOUT 3 1-CUP SERVINGS

This is the perfect smoothie for early summer when apricots are ripe. To freeze fresh apricots, cut or break them in half and remove the pits, then layer them loosely in airtight containers or freezer bags. They will keep for six months to a year. You can also drain and freeze water-packed canned apricots for this smoothie. To freeze bananas, peel them, then cut or break into 1-inch pieces. Pack loosely in airtight containers or freezer bags.

1 cup frozen banana pieces
1 cup frozen apricot halves
¼ cup apple juice concentrate

¾ cup fortified soy milk or rice milk

Combine all ingredients in a blender and process until smooth. Serve immediately.

Per 1-cup serving: 129 calories; 3 g protein; 28 g carbohydrate; 2 g fat; 8 g fiber; 14 mg sodium; calories from protein: 8%; calories from carbohydrates: 81%; calories from fats: 11%

● ● ●

Iced Green Tea

MAKES 6 1-CUP SERVINGS

Most markets sell a variety of green tea blends. Use your favorite to make this cool, refreshing beverage.

6   cups boiling water
6   green tea bags

fresh mint for garnishing (optional)

Combine water and tea bags in a large pot. Steep until cool, then remove tea bags.

Fill a glass with ice cubes and add tea. Garnish with fresh mint leaves if desired.

Per 1-cup serving: 0 calories; 0 g protein; 0 g carbohydrate; 0 g fat;
0 g fiber; 0.2 mg sodium; calories from protein: 0%;
calories from carbohydrates: 0%; calories from fats: 0%

● ● ●

Cranberry Apple Tea

MAKES 6 1-CUP SERVINGS

This tea is delicious hot or iced. A perfect blend of sweet, tart, and spicy flavors, it is made with Cranberry Cove Tea, a Celestial Seasonings product available in supermarkets and natural food stores.

4½ cups boiling water
8   Cranberry Cove tea bags
1   12-ounce can apple juice
    concentrate

orange or lemon slices for serving
(optional)

Combine water and tea bags in a large pot. Steep at least fifteen minutes.

Remove tea bags and add apple juice concentrate. Stir to mix.

For a hot beverage, heat until steamy. If desired, add a few orange or lemon slices as a garnish before serving.

For a cold beverage, chill thoroughly, then serve over ice. Garnish with orange or lemon slices if desired.

Per 1-cup serving: 96 calories; 0.2 g protein; 24 g carbohydrate;
0.2 g fat; 0.2 g fiber; 14 mg sodium; calories from protein: 1%;
calories from carbohydrates: 98%; calories from fats: 1%

Glossary

Foods That May Be New to You

The majority of ingredients in the recipes are common and widely available in grocery stores. A few that may be unfamiliar are described below.

agar   a sea vegetable used as a thickener and gelling agent instead of gelatin, an animal by-product. Available in natural food stores and Asian markets. Also may be called "agar agar." Agar comes in several forms, including powder and flakes. The powder is the easiest to measure and the most concentrated form of agar. If a recipe calls for agar flakes and you are using powder, you will have to adjust the amount you use as follows: for each teaspoon of powder called for in the recipe, use approximately 1½ tablespoonfuls of flakes to substitute.

apple juice concentrate   frozen concentrate for making apple juice. May be used full strength as a sweetener.

arrowroot   a natural thickener that may be substituted for cornstarch.

baked tofu   tofu that has been marinated and baked until it is very firm and flavorful. Baked tofu is usually available in a variety of flavors. Sold in natural food stores and many supermarkets (check the deli and produce sections).

Bakkon yeast   a type of nutritional yeast with a smoky flavor. Also called "torula yeast." Sold in natural food stores.

balsamic vinegar   mellow-flavored wine vinegar that makes delicious salad dressings and marinades. Available in most food stores.

barley flour   can be used in baked goods in place of part or all of the wheat flour for a light, somewhat crumbly product. Available in natural food stores and many supermarkets.

Bob's Red Mill products　whole grain flours, multigrain cereal, and baking mixes. Contact the manufacturer to locate a source near you.

>Bob's Red Mill Natural Foods, Inc.
>5209 S.E. International Way
>Milwaukee, OR 97222
>800-553-2258
>www.bobsredmill.com

Boca Burger　a low-fat vegetarian burger with a meaty taste and texture. Available in natural food stores, usually in the freezer case.

brown rice　an excellent source of protective soluble fiber as well as protein, vitamins, and minerals that are lost in milling white rice. Available in long-grain and short-grain varieties. Long-grain, which is light and fluffy, includes basmati, jasmine and other superbly flavorful varieties. Short-grain is more substantial and perfect for hearty dishes. Nutritionally there is very little difference between the two. Brown rice is sold in natural food stores and in many supermarkets.

bulgur　hard red winter wheat that has been cracked and toasted. Cooks quickly and has a delicious, nutty flavor. May be sold in supermarkets as "Ala."

carob powder　the roasted powder of the carob bean that can be used in place of chocolate in many recipes. Sold in natural food stores and some supermarkets.

couscous　although it looks like a grain, couscous is actually a very small pasta. Some natural food stores and supermarkets sell a whole wheat version. Look for it in the grain section.

date pieces　pitted, chopped dates that are coated with cornstarch to keep them from sticking together. They are sold in natural food stores and some supermarkets.

diced green chilies　refers to diced Anaheim chilies, which are mildly hot. These are available canned (Ortega is one brand) or fresh. When using fresh chilies, remove the skin by charring it under a broiler and rubbing it off once it has cooled.

Emes Jel　a natural gelling agent made from vegetable ingredients. May be combined with fruit juice to make a natural gelatin.

Fat-Free Nayonaise　a fat-free, cholesterol-free mayonnaise substitute that contains no dairy products or eggs. Sold in natural food stores and some supermarkets.

Fines Herbs　a herb blend that usually features equal parts of tarragon, parsley, and chives, and also may contain chervil. Look for it in the spice section.

garlic granules　another term for garlic powder.

Harvest Burger for Recipes　ready-to-use, ground beef substitute made from soy. Ideal for tacos, pasta sauces, and chili. Made by Green Giant (Pillsbury) and available in supermarket frozen food sections.

instant bean flakes   precooked black or pinto beans that can be quickly reconstituted with boiling water and used as a side dish, dip, sauce, or burrito filling. Fantastic Foods (707-778-7801) and Taste Adventure (Will-Pak Foods, 800-874-0883, www.tasteadventure.com) are two brands available in natural food stores and some supermarkets.

Italian Herbs   a commercially prepared mixture of Italian herbs: basil, oregano, thyme, marjoram, etc. Also may be called "Italian Seasoning." Look for it in the spice section of your market.

jicama ("hick-ama")   a crisp, slightly sweet root vegetable. Usually used raw in salads and with dips, but also may be added to stir-fries. Usually sold in the unrefrigerated area of the produce section.

kudzu ("kood-zoo")   a thickener made from the roots of the kudzu vine, which grows rampantly in the southeastern United States. It is used much like arrowroot or cornstarch and makes a creamy sauce or gel.

miso ("mee-so")   a salty fermented soybean paste used to flavor soup, sauces, and gravies. Available in light, medium, and dark varieties. The lighter-colored versions having the mildest flavor, while the dark are more robust. Sold in natural food stores and Asian markets.

nonhydrogenated margarine   margarine that does not contain hydrogenated oils. Hydrogenated oils raise blood cholesterol and can increase heart disease risk. Three brands of nonhydrogenated margarine are Earth Balance, Canoleo Soft Margarine, and Spectrum Spread.

nori ("nor-ee")   flat sheets of seaweed used for making sushi and nori rolls.

nutritional yeast   a good-tasting yeast that is richly endowed with nutrients, especially B vitamins. Certain nutritional yeasts, such as Red Star Vegetarian Support Formula Nutritional Yeast, are good sources of vitamin B_{12}. Check the label to be sure. Nutritional yeast may be added to foods for its flavor, sometimes described as "cheeselike," as well as for its nutritional value. Look for nutritional yeast in natural food stores.

Pacific Cream Flavored Sauce Base   a nondairy cream soup base made by Pacific Foods of Oregon and sold in natural food stores and many supermarkets.

potato flour   used as a thickener in sauces, puddings, and gravies. One common brand sold in natural food stores and many supermarkets is Bob's Red Mill.

prewashed salad mix, prewashed spinach   mixtures of lettuce, spinach, and other salad ingredients. Because they have been cleaned and dried, they store well and are easy to use. Several different mixes are available in the produce department of most food stores. "Spring mix" is particularly flavorful.

prune puree   may also be called "prune butter." Can be used in place of fat in baked goods. Commercial brands are WonderSlim and Lekvar. Prune baby food or pureed stewed prunes also may be used.

quinoa ("keen-wah")   a highly nutritious grain that cooks quickly and may be served as a side dish, pilaf, or salad. Sold in natural food stores.

red pepper flakes   dried, crushed chili peppers, available in the spice section or with the Mexican foods.

reduced-fat tofu   contains about a third of the fat of regular tofu. Three brands are Mori-Nu Lite, White Wave, and Tree of Life. Sold in natural food stores and supermarkets.

reduced-sodium soy sauce   also may be called "lite" soy sauce. Compare labels to find the brand with the lowest sodium content.

Rice Dream   see "rice milk."

rice flour   a thickener for sauces, puddings, and gravies. Choose white rice flour for the smoothest results. Bob's Red Mill is one common brand sold in natural food stores and many supermarkets.

rice milk   a beverage made from partially fermented rice that can be used in place of dairy milk on cereals and in most recipes. Available in natural food stores and some supermarkets.

roasted red peppers   red bell peppers that have been roasted over an open flame for a sweet, smoky flavor. Roast your own (see page 206) or purchase them already roasted, packed in water, in most grocery stores. Usually located near the pickles.

seasoned rice vinegar   a mild vinegar made from rice and seasoned with sugar and salt. Great for salad dressings and on cooked vegetables. Available in most grocery stores. Located with the vinegar or in the Asian foods section.

seitan ("say-tan")   also called "wheat meat," seitan is a high-protein, fat-free food with a meaty texture and flavor. Available in the deli case or freezer of natural food stores.

silken tofu   a smooth, delicate tofu that is excellent for sauces, cream soups, and dips. Often available in reduced-fat or "lite" versions. One popular brand, Mori-Nu, is widely available in convenient shelf-stable packaging—special packaging that may be stored without refrigeration for up to a year.

soba noodles   spaghetti-like pasta made with buckwheat flour. Has a delicious, distinctive flavor. Sold in natural food stores and in the Asian food section of some supermarkets.

sodium-free baking powder   made with potassium bicarbonate instead of sodium bicarbonate. Sold in natural food stores and some supermarkets. Featherweight is one brand.

soy milk   nondairy milk made from soybeans that can be used in recipes or as a beverage. May be sold fresh, powdered, or in convenient shelf-stable packaging. Choose calcium-fortified varieties. Available in natural food stores and supermarkets.

soy milk powder   can be used in smoothies, baked goods, or mixed with water for a beverage. Choose calcium-fortified varieties. Available in natural food stores and some supermarkets.

Spike   a seasoning mixture of vegetables and herbs. Comes in a salt-free version, as well as the original version, which contains salt. Sold in natural food stores and many supermarkets.

spreadable fruit   natural fruit preserves made of 100 percent fruit with no added sugar.

stone-ground mustard   mustard containing whole mustard seeds. Often contains horseradish.

tahini ("ta-hee-nee")   sesame seed butter. Comes in raw and toasted forms (either will work in the recipes in this book). Sold in natural food stores, ethnic grocery stores, and some supermarkets. Look for it near the peanut butter or with the natural or ethnic foods.

teff   the world's smallest whole grain. Cooks quickly and has a rich, nutty flavor. Delicious as a breakfast cereal. Sold in natural food stores.

textured vegetable protein (TVP)   meatlike ingredient made from defatted soy flour. Rehydrate with boiling water to add protein and meaty texture to sauces, chili, and stews. TVP is sold in natural food stores and in the bulk section of some supermarkets.

tofu   a mild-flavored soy food that is adaptable to many different recipes. Texture varies greatly, from very smooth "silken" tofu to very dense "extra-firm" tofu. Flavor is best when it is fresh, so check freshness date on package.

torula yeast   see "Bakkon yeast."

turbinado sugar   also called "raw sugar" because it is less processed than white sugar.

unbleached flour   white flour that has not been chemically whitened. Available in most grocery stores.

vegetable broth   ready-to-use brands include Pacific Foods, Imagine Foods, and Swanson's. Other brands available in dry form as powder or cubes. Sold in natural food stores and many grocery stores.

wasabe ("wa-sah-bee")   horseradish paste traditionally served with sushi. Sometimes sold fresh, but more commonly sold as a powder to be reconstituted. Look for it where Asian foods are sold.

whole wheat pastry flour   milled from soft spring wheat. Has the nutritional benefits of whole wheat and produces lighter-textured baked goods than regular whole wheat flour. Available in natural food stores.

Yves Veggie Cuisine   meatlike vegetarian products that are fat-free, including burgers, hot dogs, cold cuts, sausages, and Veggie Ground Round. Sold in natural food stores and many supermarkets.

Resources

PCRM's cancer Web site
www.cancerproject.org

Physicians Committee for Responsible Medicine
www.pcrm.org

For Healthy Eating While Traveling

Airplane travel
www.ivu.org/faq/travel.html

Directories on the Internet
www.vegdining.com and www.vegeats.com/restaurants

The Vegetarian Journal's Guide to Natural Foods Restaurants in the U.S. and Canada. Wayne, N.J.: Avery Publishing Group, 1998; updated every few years.

Cookbooks

Golbitz, Peter. *Tofu & Soyfoods Cookery.* Summertown, Tenn.: Book Publishing Company, 1998.

Grogan, Bryanna Clark. *20 Minutes to Dinner.* Summertown, Tenn.: Book Publishing Company, 1997.

Hagler, Louise. *Soyfoods Cookery.* Summertown, Tenn.: Book Publishing Company, 1996.

Melina, Vesanto, and Forest, Joseph. *Cooking Vegetarian.* New York: John Wiley & Sons and Scarborough, Ont.: Macmillan Canada, 1998.

Raymond, Jennifer. *The Peaceful Palate.* Summertown, Tenn.: Book Publishing Company, 1996.

Stepaniak, Joanne. *Vegan Vittles.* Summertown, Tenn.: Book Publishing Co., 1996.

Nutrition

American Dietetic Association and Dietitians of Canada. *Manual of Clinical Dietetics,* 6th Ed., 2000.

Davis, Brenda, and Melina, Vesanto. *Becoming Vegan.* Summertown, Tenn.: Book Publishing Company, 2000.

Heidrich, Ruth, Ph.D. *A Race for Life: From Cancer to The Ironman.* Offset House, Lantern Books, 2000.

Melina, Vesanto; Davis, Brenda; and Harrison, Victoria. *Becoming Vegetarian.* Summertown, Tenn.: Book Publishing Company, 1996.

References

Chapter 1: New Power against Cancer

Doll, R., and Peto, R. *The Causes of Cancer*. Oxford, Eng.: Oxford University Press, 1981.

Kellogg, John Harvey. *Herald of the Golden Age*, 1903.

Key, T. J.; Fraser, G. E.; and Thorogood, M. "Mortality in Vegetarians and Nonvegetarians: Detailed Findings from a Collaborative Analysis of Five Prospective Studies." *American Journal of Clinical Nutrition* 70 (1999): 516S–524S.

Parkin, D.; Muir, C.; Whelan, S.; Gao, Y.; Ferlay, J.; and Powell, J., eds. "Cancer Incidence in Five Continents." Volume VI, International Association of Cancer Registries, Scientific Publication 120. Lyons: International Agency for Research on Cancer, 1992.

World Cancer Research Fund and the American Institute of Cancer Research. *Food, Nutrition, and the Prevention of Cancer: A Global Perspective*. Washington, D.C.: American Institute of Cancer Research, 1997.

Chapter 2: Tracking Down the Culprits

Cadogan, J.; Eastell, R.; Jones, N.; and Barker, M. E. "Milk Intake and Bone Mineral Acquisition in Adolescent Girls: Randomised, Controlled Intervention Trial." *British Medical Journal* 315 (1997):1255–1260.

Chan, J. M.; Giovannucci, E.; Andersson, S. O., et al. "Dairy Products, Calcium, Phosphorus, Vitamin D, and Risk of Prostate Cancer." *Cancer Causes and Control* 9 (1998): 559–566.

Commoner, B.; Vithayathil, A. J.; Dolara, P.; Nair, S.; Madyastha, P.; and Cuca, G. C. "Formation of Mutagens in Beef and Beef Extract during Cooking." *Science* 201 (1978): 913–916.

Frentzel-Beyme, R., and Chang-Claude, J. "Vegetarian Diets and Colon Cancer: the German Experience." *American Journal of Clinical Nutrition* 59 (1994): 1143S–1152S.

Frentzel-Beyme, R.; Claude, J.; and Eilber, U. "Mortality among German Vegetarians: First Results after Five Years of Follow-up." *Nutrition and Cancer* 11 (1988):117–126.

Giovannucci, E.; Rimm, E. B.; Wolk, A.; et al. "Calcium and Fructose

222

Intake in Relation to Risk of Prostate Cancer." *Cancer Research* 58 (1998): 442–447.

Heaney, R. P.; McCarron, D.A.; Dawson-Hughes, B.; et al. "Dietary Changes Favorably Affect Bone Remodeling in Older Adults." *Journal of the American Dietetic Association* 99 (1999): 1228–1233.

Nagao, M.; Honda, M.; Seino, Y.; Yahagi, T.; and Sugimara, T. "Mutagenecities of Smoke Condensates and the Charred Surface of Fish and Meat." *Cancer Letters* 4-S (1977): 221–226.

Nagao, M., and Sugumira, T. "Carcinogenic Factors in Food with Relevance to Colon Cancer Development." *Mutation Research* 290 (1993): 343–351.

Nelson, R. L.; Davis, F. G.; Sutter, E.; Sobin, L. H.; Kikendall, J. W.; and Bowen, P. "Body Iron Stores and Risk of Colonic Neoplasia." *Journal of the National Cancer Institute* 86 (1994): 455–460.

Thorogood, M.; Mann, J.; Appleby, P.; and McPherson, K. "Risk of Death from Cancer and Ischaetic Heart Disease in Meat and Non-Meat-Eaters." *British Medical Journal* 308 (1994): 1667–1670.

Wandi, S.; Gandhi, R.; and Snedeker, S. "Critical Evaluation of Heptachlor and Heptachlor Epoxide's Breast Cancer Risk." 1998. www.cfe.cornell.edu/bcerf/CriticalEval/Pesticide/CE.heptachlor.pdf

Chapter 3: The Right Stuff: Getting the Nutrients You Need

American Dietetic Association and Dietitians of Canada. *Manual of Clinical Dietetics,* 6th ed. Chicago: American Dietetic Association and Dietitians of Canada, 2000.

American Institute of Cancer Research. *Stopping Cancer before It Starts.* New York: Golden Books, 1999.

Davis, B., and Melina, V. *Becoming Vegan.* Summertown, Tenn.: Book Publishing Company, 2000.

Deckelbaum, R.; Fisher, E. A.; Winston, M.; et al. "Summary of a Scientific Conference on Preventive Nutrition: Pediatrics to Geriatrics." *Circulation* 100 (1999): 450–456.

Melina, V.; Davis, B.; and Harrison, V. *Becoming Vegetarian.* Summertown, Tenn.: Book Publishing Company, 1995.

U.S. Department of Health and Human Services. *Healthy People 2010: Nutrition and Overweight Objectives.* www.Health.Gov/HealthyPeople www.health.gov/DietaryGuidelines/dga2000/DIETGD.PDF www.PCRM.org/Health/VSK/VSK9.html

Chapter 4: Cancer: Dietary Self-Defense

Adlercreutz, C. H.; Goldin, B. R.; Gorbach, S. L.; et al. "Soybean Phytoestrogen Intake and Cancer Risk." *Journal of Nutrition* 125 (1995): 757S–770S.

Allen, N. E.; Appleby, P. N.; Davey, G. K.; and Key, T. J. "Hormones and Diet: Low Insulin-like Growth Factor-I but Normal Bioavailable Androgens in Vegan Men." *British Journal of Cancer* 83 (2000): 95–97.

American Cancer Society. *Cancer Facts and Figures.* Atlanta: American Cancer Society, 1994.

American Institute of Cancer Research. *Stopping Cancer before It Starts.* New York: Golden Books, 1999.

Brigelius-Flohe, R., and Traber, M. "Vitamin E: Function and Metabolism." *The FASEB* [Federation of American Societies of Experimental Biology] *Journal* 13 (1999): 1145–1155.

Cassidy, A.; Bingham, S.; and Carlson, J. "Biological Effects of Plant Estrogens in Premenopausal Women." *The FASEB* [Federation of American Societies of Experimental Biology] *Journal* 7 (1993): A866.

Chatenoud, L.; La Vecchia, C.; Franceschi, S.; et al. "Refined-Cereal Intake and Risk of Selected Cancers in Italy." *American Journal of Clinical Nutrition* 70 (1999): 1107–1110.

Chu, S. Y.; Lee, N. C.; Wingo, P. A.; Senie, R. T.; Greenberg, R. S.; and Peterson, H. B. "The Relationship between Body Mass and Breast Cancer among Women Enrolled in the Cancer and Steroid Hormone Study." *Journal of Clinical Epidemiology* 44 (1991): 1197–1206.

Craig, W. *Nutrition and Wellness.* New York: Golden Harvest Books, 1999.

De Ridder, C. M.; Thijssen, J. H.; Van 't Veer, P.; et al. "Dietary Habits, Sexual Maturation, and Plasma Hormones in Pubertal Girls: A Longitudinal Study." *American Journal of Clinical Nutrition* 54 (1991): 805–813.

Gaard, M.; Tretli, S.; and Loken, E. B. "Dietary Fat and the Risk of Breast Cancer: A Prospective Study of 25,892 Norwegian Women." *International Journal of Cancer* 63 (1995): 13–17.

Garabrant, D. H.; Peters, J. M.; Mack, T. M.; and Bernstein, L. "Job Activity and Colon Cancer Risk." *American Journal of Epidemiology* 119 (1984): 1005–1014.

Giovannucci, E.; Ascherio, A.; Rimm, E. B.; Stampfer, M. J.; Colditz, G. A.; and Willett, W. C. "Intake of Carotenoids and Retinol in Relation to Risk of Prostate Cancer." *Journal of the National Cancer Institute* 87 (1995): 1767–1776.

Goldin, B. R.; Adlercreutz, H.; Gorbach, S. L.; et al. Estrogen Excretion Patterns and Plasma Levels in Vegetarian and Omnivorous Women." *New England Journal of Medicine* 307 (1982): 1542–1547.

Goodman, M. T.; Hankin, J. H.; Wilkens, L. R.; and Kolonel, L. N. "High-Fat Foods and the Risk of Lung Cancer." *Epidemiology* 3 (1992): 288–299.

Grant, W. B. "An Ecologic Study of Dietary Links to Prostate Cancer." *Alternative Medicine Review* 4, no. 3 (1999): 162–169.

Haenszel, W.; Berg, J.; Segi, M.; Kurihara, M.; and Locke, F. B. "Large Bowel Cancer in Hawaiian Japanese." *Journal of the National Cancer Institute* 51 (1973): 1765–1779.

Heber, D. "What's New in Diet and Cancer Prevention." Denver: American Dietetic Association Convention, October 16–19, 2000.

Jansen, M. C.; Bueno-de-Mesquita, H. B.; Buzina, R.; et al. "Dietary Fiber and Plant Foods in Relation to Colorectal Cancer Mortality: The Seven Countries Study." *International Journal of Cancer* 81 (1999): 174–179.

Kolonel, L. N.; Hankin, J. H.; Whittemore, A. S.; et al. "Vegetables, Fruits, Legumes and Prostate Cancer: A Multiethnic Case-Control Study." *Cancer, Epidemiology, Biomarkers, and Prevention* 9 (2000): 795–804.

Kromhout, D. "Essential Micronutrients in Relation to Carcinogenesis." American Journal of *Clinical Nutrition* 45 (1987): 1361–1367.

Lee, H. P.; Gourley, L.; Duffy, S.W.; Esteve, J.; Lee, J.; and Day, N. E. "Dietary Effects on Breast-Cancer Risk in Singapore." *Lancet* 337 (1991): 1197–1200.

Lu, L. J.; Anderson, K. E.; Grady, J. J.; and Nagamani, M. "Effects of Soya Consumption for One Month on Steroid Hormones in Premenopausal Women: Implications for Breast Cancer Risk Reduction." *Cancer, Epidemiology, Biomarkers, and Prevention* 5 (1996): 63–70.

McCarty, M. F. "Vegan Proteins May Reduce Risk of Cancer, Obesity, and Cardiovascular Disease by Promoting Increased Glucagon Activity." *Medical Hypotheses* 53 (1999): 459–485.

Messina, M. J. "Legumes and Soybeans: Overview of Their Nutritional Profiles and Health Effects." *American Journal of Clinical Nutrition* 70 (1999): 439S–450S.

Messina, M. J.; Persky, V.; Setchell, K. D.; and Barnes, S. "Soy Intake and Cancer Risk: A Review of the In Vitro and In Vivo Data." *Nutrition and Cancer* 21 (1994): 113–131.

Michnovicz, J. J., and Bradlow, H. L. "Induction of Estradiol Metabolism by Dietary Indole-3-Carbinol in Humans." *Journal of the National Cancer Institute* 82 (1990): 947–949.

Mills, P. K.; Beeson, W. L.; Phillips, R. L.; and Fraser, G. E. "Cohort Study of Diet, Lifestyle, and Prostate Cancer in Adventist Men." *Cancer* 64 (1989): 598–604.

Nelson, R. L.; Davis, F. G.; Sutter, E.; Sobin, L. H.; Kikendall, J. W.; and Bowen, P. "Body Iron Stores and Risk of Colonic Neoplasia." *Journal of the National Cancer Institute* 86 (1994): 455–460.

Patterson, B. H.; Block, G.; Rosenberger, W. F.; Pee, D.; and Kahle, L. L. "Fruit and Vegetables in the American Diet: Data from the NHANES II Survey." *American Journal of Public Health* 80 (1990): 1443–1449.

Persky, V. W.; Chatterton, R. T.; Van Horn, L. V.; Grant, M. D.; Langenberg, P.; and Marvin, J. "Hormone Levels in Vegetarian and Nonvegetarian Teenage Girls: Potential Implications for Breast Cancer Risk." *Cancer Research* 52 (1992): 578–583.

Prentice, R.L.; Kakar, F.; Hursting, S.; Sheppard, L.; Klein, R.; and Kushi, L. H. "Aspects of the Rationale for the Women's Health Trial." *Journal of the National Cancer Institute* 80 (1988): 802–814.

Roberts-Thompson, I.; Ryan, P.; Khoo, K.; Hart, W.; McMichael, A.; and Butler, R. "Diet, Acetylator Phenotype, and Risk of Colorectal Neoplasia." *Lancet* 347 (1996): 1372–1373.

Slavin, J. L. "Mechanisms for the Impact of Whole Grain Foods on Cancer Risk." *Journal of the American College of Nutrition* 19 (2000): 300S–307S

Slavin, J. L.; Martini, M. C.; Jacobs, D. R. Jr.; and Marquart, L. "Plausible Mechanisms for the Protectiveness of Whole Grains." *American Journal of Clinical Nutrition* 70 (1999): 459S–463S.

Steinmetz, K. A., and Potter, J. D. "Vegetables, Fruit, and Cancer I: Epidemiology." *Cancer Causes and Control* 2 (1991): 325–357.

———. "Vegetables, Fruit, and Cancer II: Mechanisms." *Cancer Causes and Control* 2 (1991): 427–442.

Stephens, F. O. "Breast Cancer: Aetiological Factors and Associations (a Possible Protective Role of Phytoestrogens)." *Australian and New Zealand Journal of Surgery* 67 (1997): 755–760.

Tamir, S.; Eizenberg, M.; Somjen, D.; et al. "Estrogenic and Antiproliferative Properties of Glabridin from Licorice in Human Breast Cancer Cells." *Cancer Research* 60 (2000): 5704–5709.

Thompson, L. "Potential Health Benefits of Whole Grains and Their Components." *Contemporary Nutrition* 17 (1992): 1–2.

Thun, M.; Calle, E.; Namboodiri, M.; et al. "Risk Factors for Fatal Colon Cancer in a Large Prospective Study." *Journal of the National Cancer Institute* 84 (1992): 1491–1500.

Toniolo, P.; Riboli, E.; Protta, F.; Charrel, M.; and Cappa, A. P. "Calorie-Providing Nutrients and Risk of Breast Cancer." *Journal of the National Cancer Institute* 81 (1989): 278–286.

Toniolo, P.; Riboli, E.; Shore, R. E.; and Pasternack, B. S. "Consumption of Meat, Animal Products, Protein, and Fat and Risk of Breast Cancer: A Prospective Cohort Study in New York." *Epidemiology* 5 (1994): 391–397.

Trichopoulou, A.; Katsouyanni, K.; Stuver, S.; et al. "Consumption of Olive Oil and Specific Food Groups in Relation to Breast Cancer Risk in Greece." *Journal of the National Cancer Institute* 87 (1995): 110–116.

Trock, B.; Lanza, E.; and Greenwald, P. "Dietary Fiber, Vegetables, and Colon Cancer: Critical Review and Meta-Analyses of the Epidemiologic Evidence." *Journal of the National Cancer Institute* 82 (1990): 650–661.

Watson, R. R.; Prabhala, R. H.; Plezia, P. M.; and Alberts, D. S. "Effect of Beta-Carotene on Lymphocyte Subpopulations in Elderly Humans: Evidence for a Dose-Response Relationship." *American Journal of Clinical Nutrition* 53 (1991): 988.

West, D. W.; Slattery, M. L.; Robison, L. M.; French, T. K.; and Mahoney, A. W. "Adult Dietary Intake and Prostate Cancer Risk in Utah: A Case-Control Study with Special Emphasis on Aggressive Tumors." *Cancer Causes and Control* 2 (1991): 85–94.

World Cancer Research Fund and the American Institute of Cancer Research. *Food, Nutrition, and the Prevention of Cancer: A Global Perspective.* Washington, D.C.: American Institute of Cancer Research, 1997.

Wu, A.; Malcolm, C.; and Pike, D. O. "Stram Meta-Analysis: Dietary Fat Intake, Serum Estrogen Levels, and the Risk of Breast Cancer." *Journal of the National Cancer Institute* 91 (1999): 529–534.

Ziegler, R. G. "Vegetables, Fruits, and Carotenoids and the Risk of Cancer." *American Journal of Clinical Nutrition* 53 (1991): 251S–259S.

Chapter 5: Foods for Cancer Survival

Baehner, R. L.; Boxer, L. A.; Ingraham, L. M.; Butterick, C.; and Haak, R. A. "The Influence of Vitamin E on Human Polymorphonuclear Cell Metabolism and Function." *Annals of the New York Academy of Sciences* 393 (1981): 237–249.

Barnard, N. D.; Scialli, A. R.; Hurlock, D.; and Bertron, P. "Diet and Sex-Hormone Binding Globulin, Dysmenorrhea, and Premenstrual Symptoms." *Obstetrics and Gynecology* 95 (2000): 245–250.

Baron, J.; Hebert, J. R.; and Reddy, M.M. "Dietary Factors and Natural-Killer-Cell Activity." *American Journal of Clinical Nutrition* 50 (1989): 861–867.

Cuthbert, J. A., and Lipsky, P. E. "Immunoregulation by Low Density Lipoproteins in Man." *Journal of Clinical Investigation* 73 (1984): 992–1003.

DeCosse, J. J.; Miller, H. H.; and Lesser, M. L. "Effect of Wheat Fiber and Vitamins C and E on Rectal Polyps in Patients with Familial Adenomatous Polyposis." *Journal of the National Cancer Institute* 81 (1989): 1290–1297.

Engle, W. A.; Yoder, M. C.; Baurley, J. L.; and Poa-Lo, Y. U. "Vitamin E Decreases Superoxide Anion Production by Polymorphonuclear Leukocytes." *Pediatric Research* 23 (1988): 245–248.

Garewal, H. S.; Katz, R. V.; Meyskens, F.; et al. Beta-Carotene Produces Sustained Remissions in Patients with Oral Leukoplakia." *Archives of Otolaryngological Head and Neck Surgery* 125 (1999): 1305–1310.

Gregorio, D. I.; Emrich, L. J.; Graham, S.; Marshall, J. R.; and Nemoto, T. "Dietary Fat Consumption and Survival among Women with Breast Cancer." *Journal of the National Cancer Institute* 75 (1985): 37–41.

Hawley, H. P., and Gordon, G. B. "The Effects of Long-Chain Free Fatty Acids on Human Neutrophil Function and Structure." *Laboratory Investigation* 34 (1976): 216–222.

Heaney, R. P.; McCarron, D. A.; Dawson-Hughes, B.; et al. "Dietary Changes Favorably Affect Bone Remodeling in Older Adults." *Journal of the American Dietetic Association* 99 (1999): 1228–1233.

Kim, Y. I. "AGA Technical Review: Impact of Dietary Fiber on Colon Cancer Occurrence." *Gastroenterology* 118 (2000): 1235–1257.

Meydani, S. N.; Meydani, M.; Barklund, P. M.; et al. "Effect of Vitamin E Supplementation on Immune Responsiveness of the Aged." *Annals of the New York Academy of Sciences* 570 (1989): 283–290.

Nakachi, K.; Suemasu, K.; Suga, K.; Takeo, T.; Imai, K.; and Higashi, Y. "Influence of Drinking Green Tea on Breast Cancer Malignancy among Japanese Patients." *Japanese Journal of Cancer Research* 89 (1998): 254–261.

Nordenstrom, J.; Jarstran, C.; and Wiernik, A. "Decreased Chemotactic and Random Migration of Leukocytes during Intralipid Infusion." *American Journal of Clinical Nutrition* 32 (1979): 2416–2422.

Pepe, M. G., and Curtiss, L. K. "Apolipoprotein E is a Biologically Active Constituent of the Normal Immunoregulatory Lipoprotein LDL-In." *Journal of Immunology* 136 (1986): 3716–3723.

Prasad, J. S. "Effect of Vitamin E Supplementation on Leukocyte Function." *American Journal of Clinical Nutrition* 33 (1980): 606–608.

Prentice, R.; Thompson, D.; Clifford, C.; Gorbach, S.; Goldin, B.; and Byar, D. "Dietary Fat Reduction and Plasma Estradiol Concentration in Healthy Postmenopausal Women." *Journal of the National Cancer Institute* 82 (1990): 129–134.

Saxe, G. A.; Rock, C. L.; Wicha, M. S.; and Schottenfeld, D. "Diet and Risk for Breast Cancer Recurrence and Survival." *Breast Cancer Research and Treatment* 53 (1999): 241–253.

Schapira, D. V.; Kumar, N. B.; Lyman, G. H.; and Cox, C.E. "Obesity and Body Fat Distribution and Breast Cancer Prognosis." *Cancer* 67 (1991): 523–528.

Traill, K. N.; Huber, L. A.; Wick, G.; and Jurgens, G. "Lipoprotein Interactions with T Cells: An Update." *Immunology* 11 (1990): 411–417.

Verreault, R.; Brisson, J.; Deschenes, L.; Naud, F.; Meyer, F.; and Belanger, L. "Dietary Fat in Relation to Prognostic Indicators in Breast Cancer." *Journal of the National Cancer Institute* 80 (1988): 819–825.

Watson, R. R.; Prabhala, R. H.; Plezia, P. M.; and Alberts, D. S. "Effect of Beta-Carotene on Lymphocyte Subpopulations in Elderly Humans: Evidence for a Dose-Response Relationship." *American Journal of Clinical Nutrition* 53 (1991): 90–94.

Wynder, E. L.; Kajitani, T.; Kuno, J.; Lucas, J. C. Jr.; DePalo, A.; and Farrow, J. "A Comparison of Survival Rates between American and Japanese Patients with Breast Cancer." *Surgical Gynecology and Obstetrics* 117 (1963): 196–200.

Zhang, S.; Folsom, A. R.; Sellers, T. A.; Kushi, L. H.; and Potter, J. D. "Better Breast Cancer Survival for Postmenopausal Women Who Are Less Overweight and Eat Less Fat." *Cancer* 76 (1995): 275–283.

Chapter 6: Nutrition during Cancer Treatment

American Cancer Society Workgroup on Nutrition and Physical Activity for Cancer Survivors. "Nutrition during and after Cancer Treatment." American Dietetic Association Convention, October 18, 2000, Denver.

American Dietetic Association and Dietitians of Canada. *Manual of Clinical Dietetics,* 6th ed. Chicago: American Dietetic Association, 2000.

Barone, J.; Hebert, J.; and Reddy, M. "Dietary Fat and Natural-Killer-Cell Activity." *American Journal of Clinical Nutrition* 50 (1989): 861–867.

Block Medical Center. www.BlockMD.com

Bub, A.; Watzl, B.; Abrahamse, L.; et al. "Moderate Intervention with

Carotenoid-Rich Vegetable Products Reduces Lipid Peroxidation in Men." *Journal of Nutrition* 130 (2000): 2200–2206.

Cohen, L. A.; Rose, D. P.; and Wydner, E. L. "A Rationale for Dietary Intervention in Postmenopausal Breast Cancer Patients: An Update." *Nutrition and Cancer* 19 (1993): 1–10.

Gregorio, D. I.; Emrich, L. J.; Graham, S.; Marshall, J. R.; and Nemoto, T. "Dietary Fat Consumption and Survival among Women with Breast Cancer." *Journal of the National Cancer Institute* 75 (1985): 37–41.

Haddad, E. H.; Berk, L. S.; Kettering, J. D.; Hubbard, R. W.; and Peters, W. R. "Dietary Intake and Biochemical, Hematologic, and Immune Status of Vegans Compared with Nonvegetarians." *American Journal of Clinical Nutrition* 70 (1999): 586–593.

Hebert, J. R., and Toporoff, E. "Dietary Exposures and Other Factors of Possible Prognostic Significance in Relation to Tumour Size and Nodal Involvement in Early-Stage Breast Cancer." *International Journal of Epidemiology* 18 (1989): 518–526.

Holm, L. E.; Nordevang, E.; Hjalmar, M. L.; Lidbrink, E.; Callmer, E.; and Nilsson, B. "Treatment Failure and Dietary Habits in Women with Breast Cancer." *Journal of the National Cancer Instiitute* 85 (1993): 32–36.

Hsieh, T. C., and Wu, J. M. "Cell Growth and Gene Modulatory Activities of Yunzhi (Windsor Wunxi) from Mushroom Trametes Versicolor in Androgen-Dependent and Androgen-Insensitive Human Prostate Cancer Cells." *International Journal of Oncology* 18 (2001): 81–88.

Imoberdorf, R. "Immuno-Nutrition: Designer Diets in Cancer." *Support Care Cancer* 5 (1997): 381–386.

Ingram, D. M.; Roberts, A.; and Nottage, E. M. "Host Factors and Breast Cancer Growth Characteristics." *European Journal of Cancer* 28A (1992): 1153–1161.

Kradjian, Robert M. www.newveg.av.org/health/kradjian.htm

MacLennan, R.; Macrae, F.; Bain, C.; et al. "Randomized Trial of Intake of Fat, Fiber, and Beta-Carotene to Prevent Colorectal Adenomas. The Australian Polyp Prevention Project." *Journal of the National Cancer Institute* 87 (1995): 1760–1766.

Macrae, F. "Wheat Bran Fiber and Development of Adenomatous Polyps: Evidence from Randomized, Controlled Clinical Trials." *American Journal of Medicine* 106 (1999): 38S–42S.

McCarty, M. "Vegan Proteins May Reduce Risk of Cancer, Obesity, and Cardiovascular Disease by Promoting Increased Glucagon Activity." *Medical Hypotheses* 53 (1999): 459–485.

Messina, M. "Soy, Soy Phytoestrogens (Isoflavones), and Breast Cancer" (letter). *American Journal of Clinical Nutrition* 70 (1999): 574–575.

Messina, M. J. "Legumes and Soybeans: Overview of Their Nutritional Profiles and Health Effects." *American Journal of Clinical Nutrition* 70 (1999): 439S–450S.

Messina, M., and Messina, V. *The Dietitian's Guide to Vegetarian Diets.* Gaithersburg, Md.: Aspen, 1996.

Michnovicz, J. J., and Bradlow, H. L. "Induction of Estradiol Metabolism by Dietary Indole-3-Carbinol in Humans." *Journal of the National Cancer Institute* 82 (1990): 947–949.

Nomura, A. M.; Marchand, L. L.; Kolonel, L. N.; and Hankin, J. H. "The Effect of Dietary Fat on Breast Cancer Survival among Caucasians and Japanese Women in Hawaii." *Breast Cancer Research and Treatment* 18 (1991): 135S –141S.

Perez, C., and Brady, L. *Principles and Practice of Radiation Oncology,* 3rd ed. Philadelphia: Lippincott-Raven, 1998.

Perlmutter, D. *A Quarterly Health Update,* 1, no. 3 (1996). www.perlhealth.com

Peterson, G., and Barnes, S. "Genistein and Biochanin A Inhibit Growth of Human Prostate Cancer Cells but Not Epidermal Growth Factor Receptor Tyrosine Autophosphorylation." *The Prostate* 22 (1993): 335–345.

Review. "Nutritional Therapies: Questionable Methods of Cancer Management." *CA Cancer J Clin* 43 (1993): 309–319.

Rose, D. P. "Dietary Fat, Fatty Acids, and Breast Cancer." *Breast Cancer* 4 (1997): 7–16.

Saxe, G. A.; Rock, C. L.; Wicha, M. S.; and Schottenfeld, D. "Diet and Risk for Breast Cancer Recurrence and Survival." *Breast Cancer Research and Treatment* 53 (1999): 241–253.

Verhagen, H.; Rauma, A. L.; and Torronen, R. "Effect of a Vegan Diet on Biomarkers of Chemoprevention in Females." *Human and Experimental Toxicology* 15 (1996): 821–825.

Weitzman, S. "Alternative Nutritional Cancer Therapies." *International Journal of Cancer Supplement* 11 (1998): 69–72.

Chapter 7: Putting Food Power to Work against Today's Common Cancers

General

World Cancer Research Fund and American Institute for Cancer Research. *Food, Nutrition, and the Prevention of Cancer: A Global Perspective.* Washington, D.C.: American Institute for Cancer Research, 1997.

Lung

Albanes, D. "Beta-Carotene and Lung Cancer: A Case Study." *American Journal of Clinical Nutrition* 69 (1999): 1345S–1350S.

Block, G.; Patterson, B.; and Subar, A. "Fruit, Vegetables, and Cancer Prevention: A Review of the Epidemiological Evidence." *Nutrition and Cancer* 18 (1992): 1–29.

Candelora, E. C.; Stockwell, H. G.; Armstrong, A. W.; et al. "Dietary Intake and Risk of Lung Cancer in Women Who Never Smoked." *Nutrition and Cancer* 17 (1992): 263–270.

Goodman, M. T.; Kolonel, L. N.; Wilkens, L. R.; et al. "Dietary Factors in Lung Cancer Prognosis." *European Journal of Cancer* 28 (1992): 495–501.

Mulder, I.; Jansen, M. C.; Smit, H. A.; et al. "Role of Smoking and Diet in the Cross-Cultural Variation in Lung-Cancer Mortality: The Seven Countries Study." *International Journal of Cancer* 88 (2000): 665–671.

Shibata, A.; Paganini-Hill, A.; Ross, R. K.; et al. "Dietary Beta-Carotene, Cigarette Smoking, and Lung Cancer in Men." *Cancer Causes and Control* 3 (1992): 207–214.

Steinmetz, K.A.; Potter, J. D.; and Folsom, A. R. "Vegetables, Fruit, and Lung Cancer in the Iowa Women's Health Study." *Cancer Research* 53 (1993): 536–543.

Prostate

Allen, N. E.; Appleby, P. N.; Davey, G. K.; et al. "Hormones and Diet: Low Insulin-Like Growth Factor-I but Normal Bioavailable Androgens in Vegan Men." *British Journal of Cancer* 83 (2000): 95–97.

Cadogan, J.; Eastell, R.; Jones, N.; et al. "Milk Intake and Bone Mineral Acquisition in Adolescent Girls: Randomised, Controlled Intervention Trial." *British Medical Journal* 315 (1997): 1255–1260.

Chan, J.; Stampfer, M. J.; and Giovannucci, E. L. "What Causes Prostate Cancer? A Brief Summary of the Epidemiology." *Seminars in Cancer Biology* 8 (1998): 263–273.

Cohen, P. "Serum Insulin-Like Growth Factor-I Levels and Prostate Cancer Risk—Interpreting the Evidence." *Journal of the National Cancer Institute* 90 (1998): 876–879.

Giovannucci, E. "Dietary Influences of 1,25(OH)$_2$ Vitamin D in Relation to Prostate Cancer: A Hypothesis." *Cancer Causes and Control* 9 (1998): 567–582.

Heaney, R. P.; McCarron, D. A.; Dawson-Hughes, B.; et al. "Dietary Changes Favorably Affect Bone Remodeling in Older Adults." *Journal of the American Dietetic Association* 99 (1999): 1228–1233.

Jacobsen, B. K.; Knutsen, S. F.; and Fraser, G. E. "Does High Soy Milk Intake Reduce Prostate Cancer Incidence?" The Adventist Health Study (United States). *Cancer Causes and Control* 9 (1998): 553–557.

Kontessis, P. S.; Trevisan, R.; Bossinakou, I.; et al. "Renal, Metabolic, and Hormonal Responses to Proteins of Different Origin in Normotensive, Nonproteinuric Type I Diabetic Patients." *Diabetes Care* 18 (1995): 1233–1240.

Severson, R. K.; Nomura, A. M. Y.; Grove, J. S.; et al. "A Prospective Study of Demographics, Diet, and Prostate Cancer among Men of Japanese Ancestry in Hawaii." *Cancer Research* 49 (1989): 1857–1860.

Breast

Ingram, D. M.; Roberts, A.; and Nottage, E. M. "Host Factors and Breast Cancer Growth Characteristics." *European Journal of Cancer* 28A (1992): 1153–1161.

Colon

Graham, S.; Dayal, H.; Swanson, M.; et al. "Diet in the Epidemiology of Cancer of the Colon and Rectum." *Journal of the National Cancer Institute* 61 (1978): 709–714.

Thun, M. J.; Calle, E. E.; Namboodiri, M. M.; et al. "Risk Factors for Fatal Colon Cancer in a Large Prospective Study." *Journal of the National Cancer Institute* 84 (1992): 1491–1500.

Ovarian

Casagrande, J. T.; Pike, M. C.; and Henderson, B. E. "Oral Contraceptives and Ovarian Cancer." *New England Journal of Medicine* 308 (1983): 843–844.

Kerber, R. A., and Slattery, M. L. "The Impact of Family History on Ovarian Cancer Risk. The Utah Population Database." *Archives of Internal Medicine* 155 (1995): 905–912.

Rose, D. P.; Boyar, A. P.; and Wynder, E. L. "International Comparisons of Mortality Rates for Cancer of the Breast, Ovary, Prostate, and Colon, and Per Capita Food Consumption." *Cancer* 58 (1986): 2363–2371.

Cervical

Albanes, D.; Blair, A.; and Taylor, P. R. "Physical Activity and Risk of Cancer in the NHANES 1 Population." *American Journal of Public Health* 79 (1989): 744–750.

Frisch, R. E.; Wyshak, G.; and Albright, N. L. "Former Athletes Have a Lower Lifetime Occurrence of Breast Cancer and Cancers of the Reproductive System." *Advances in Experimental Medicine and Biology* 322 (1992): 29–39.

Verrault, R.; Chu, J.; Mandelson, M.; and Shy, K. "A Case-Control Study of Diet and Invasive Cervical Cancer." *International Journal of Cancer* 43 (1989): 1050–1054.

Ziegler, R. G.; Jones, C. J.; Brinton, L. A.; et al. "Diet and Risk of In Situ Cervical Cancer among White Women in the United States." *Cancer Causes and Control* 2 (1991): 17–29.

Chapter 8: Treating Yourself to Good Food and Great Health

American Institute of Cancer Research. *Stopping Cancer before It Starts.* New York: Golden Books, 1999.

Broadbent, T. A., and Broadbent, H. S. "The Chemistry and Pharmacology of Indole-3-Carbinol (Indole-3-Methanol) and 3-(Methoxymethyl)Indole." *Current Medicinal Chemistry* 5 (1998): 469–491.

Castellsague, X.; Munoz, N.; De Stefani, E.; Victora, C. G.; Castelletto, R.; and Rolon, P. A. "Influence of Mate Drinking, Hot Beverages, and Diet on Esophageal Cancer Risk in South America." *International Journal of Cancer* 88 (2000): 658–664.

Consumers Union, nonprofit publisher of *Consumer Reports* magazine www.consumersunion.org/food/food.htm#pesticides

Gartner, C.; Stahl, W.; and Sies, H. "Lycopene is More Bioavailable from Tomato Paste Than from Fresh Tomatoes." *American Journal of Clinical Nutrition* 66 (1997): 116–122.

Hanninen, O.; Rauma, A. L.; Kaartinen, K.; and Nenonen, M. "Vegan Diet and Bacterial Enzymes." *Acta Physiologica Hungarica* 86 (1999): 171–180.

Kuper, H.; Titus-Ernstoff, L.; Harlow, B. L.; and Cramer, D. W. "Population-Based Study of Coffee, Alcohol, and Tobacco Use and Risk of Ovarian Cancer." *International Journal of Cancer* 88 (2000): 313–318.

Ling, W. H., and Hanninen, O. "Shifting from a Conventional Diet to an Uncooked Vegan Diet Reversibly Alters Fecal Hydrolytic Activities in Humans." *Journal of Nutrition* 122 (1992): 924–930.

Meinert, R.; Schuz, J.; Kaletsch, U.; Kaatsch, P.; and Michaelis, J. "Leukemia and Non-Hodgkin's Lymphoma in Childhood and Exposure to Pesticides: Results of a Register-Based Case-Control Study in Germany." *American Journal of Epidemiology* 151 (2000): 639–650.

Mukhtar, H., and Ahmad, N. "Tea Polyphenols: Prevention of Cancer and Optimizing Health." *American Journal of Clinical Nutrition* 71 (2000): 1698S–1702S.

Talcott, S. T.; Howard, L. R.; and Brenes, C. H. "Antioxidant Changes and Sensory Properties of Carrot Puree Processed with and without Periderm Tissue." *Journal of Agriculture and Food Chemistry* 48 (2000): 1315–1321.

World Cancer Research Fund and American Institute of Cancer Research. *Food, Nutrition, and the Prevention of Cancer: A Global Perspective.* Washington, D.C.: American Institute of Cancer Research, 1997.

Chapter 9: Fitness, Friendship, and Freedom from Stress

Bernstein, L.; Henderson, B. E.; Hanisch, R.; Sullivan-Halley, J.; and Ross, R. K. "Physical Exercise and Reduced Risk of Breast Cancer in Young Women." *Journal of the National Cancer Institute* 86 (1994): 1403–1408.

Butow, P. N.; Hiller, J. E.; Price, M. A.; Thackway, S.; Kricker, A.; and Tennant, C. C. "Epidemiological Evidence for a Relationship between Life Events, Coping Style, and Personality Factors in the Development of Breast Cancer." *Journal of Psychosomatic Research* 49 (2000): 169–181.

Coker, K. H. "Meditation and Prostate Cancer: Integrating a Mind/Body Intervention with Traditional Therapies." *Seminars in Urologic Oncology* 17 (1999): 111–118.

Colditz, G. A., and Rosner, B. "Cumulative Risk of Breast Cancer to Age 70 Years According to Risk Factor Status: Data from the Nurses' Health Study." *American Journal of Epidemiology* 152 (2000): 950–964.

Courneya, K. S.; Keats, M. R.; and Turner, A. R. "Physical Exercise and Quality of Life in Cancer Patients Following High Dose Chemotherapy and Autologous Bone Marrow Transplantation." *Psychooncology* 9 (2000): 127–136.

Cunningham, A. J.; Phillips, C.; Lockwood, G. A.; Hedley, D. W.; and Edmonds, C. V. "Association of Involvement in Psychological Self-Regulation with Longer Survival in Patients with Metastatic Cancer: An Exploratory Study." *Advances in Mind-Body Medicine* 16 (2000): 276–287.

Czyzyk, A., and Szczepanik, Z. "Diabetes Mellitus and Cancer." *European Journal of Internal Medicine* 11 (2000): 245–252.

Dimeo, F. "Exercise for Cancer Patients: A New Challenge in Sports Medicine." *Western Journal of Medicine* 173 (2000): 272–273.

Fredette, S. L. "Breast Cancer Survivors: Concerns and Coping." *Cancer Nursing* 18 (1995): 35–46.

Garabrant, D. H.; Peters, J. M.; Mack, T. M.; and Bernstein, L. "Job Activity and Colon Cancer Risk." *American Journal of Epidemiology* 119 (1984): 1005–1014.

Gerits, P., and De Brabander, B. "Psychosocial Predictors of Psychological, Neurochemical, and Immunological Symptoms of Acute Stress among Breast Cancer Patients." *Psychiatry Research* 85 (1999): 95–103.

Giovannucci, E.; Leitzmann, M.; Spiegelman, D.; et al. "A Prospective Study of Physical Activity and Prostate Cancer in Male Health Professionals." *Cancer Research* 58 (1998): 5117–5122.

Kavan, M. G.; Engdahl, B. E.; and Kay, S. "Colon Cancer: Personality Factors Predictive of Onset and Stage of Presentation." *Journal of Psychosomatic Research* 39 (1995): 1031–1039.

Lee, I. M.; Paffenbarger, R. S. Jr.; and Hsieh, C. "Physical Activity and Risk of Developing Colorectal Cancer among College Alumni." *Journal of the National Cancer Institute* 83 (1991): 1324–1329.

McKenna, M. C.; Zevon, M. A.; Corn, B.; and Rounds, J. "Psychosocial Factors and the Development of Breast Cancer: A Meta-Analysis." *Health Psychology* 18 (1999): 520–531.

McTiernan, A. "Physical Activity and the Prevention of Breast Cancer." *Medscape Women's Health* 5 (2000): E1.

Moradi, T.; Nyren, O.; Zack, M.; Magnusson, C.; Persson, I.; and Adami, H. O. "Breast Cancer Risk and Lifetime Leisure-Time and Occupational Physical Activity (Sweden)." *Cancer Causes and Control.* 11 (2000): 523–531.

Moradi, T.; Weiderpass, E.; Signorello, L. B.; Persson, I.; Nyren, O.; and Adami, H. O. "Physical Activity and Postmenopausal Endometrial Cancer Risk." *Cancer Causes and Control* 11 (2000): 829–837.

Murphy, T. K.; Calle, E. E.; Rodriguez, C.; Khan, H. S.; and Thun, M. J. "Body Mass Index and Colon Cancer Mortality in a Large Prospective Study." *American Journal of Epidemiology* 152 (2000): 847–854.

Pinnock, C. B.; Stapleton, A. M.; and Marshall, V. R. "Erectile Dysfunction in the Community: A Prevalence Study." *Medical Journal of Australia* 171 (1999): 353–257.

Porock, D.; Kristjanson, L. J.; Tinnelly, K.; Duke, T.; and Blight, J. "An Exercise Intervention for Advanced Cancer Patients Experiencing Fatigue: A Pilot Study." *Journal of Palliative Care* 16 (2000): 30–36.

Remen, R. N. *Kitchen Table Wisdom,* 1996.

Rosenbaum, E. H., and Rosenbaum, I. *Cancer Supportive Care: A Comprehensive Guide for Patients and Their Families.* Toronto: Somerville House Books, 1998.

Sandler, R. S. "Prevention of Colorectal Cancer." *Current Treatment Options in Gastroenterology* 2 (1999): 27–33.

Schwartz, A. L. "Daily Fatigue Patterns and Effect of Exercise in Women with Breast Cancer." *Cancer Practice* 8 (2000): 16–24.

Siegel, B. S. *How to Live between Office Visits.* New York: HarperCollins Audio, 1993.

Simon, H. "The Immunology of Exercise: A Brief Review." *Journal of the American Medical Association* 252 (1984): 2735–2738.

Slattery, M. L. "Diet, Lifestyle, and Colon Cancer." *Seminars in Gastrointestinal Disease* 11 (2000): 142–146.

Slattery, M. L.; Edwards, S. L.; Ma, K. N.; Friedman, G. D.; and Potter, J. D. "Physical Activity and Colon Cancer: A Public Health Perspective." *Annals of Epidemiology* 7 (1997): 137–145.

Speca, M.; Carlson, L. E.; Goodey, E.; and Angen, M. "A Randomized, Wait-List Controlled Clinical Trial: The Effect of a Mindfulness Meditation-Based Stress Reduction Program on Mood and Symptoms of Stress in Cancer Outpatients." *Psychosomatic Medicine* 62 (2000): 613–622.

Verloop, J.; Rookus, M. A.; van der Kooy, K.; and van Leeuwen, F. E. "Physical Activity and Breast Cancer Risk in Women Aged 20–54 Years." *Journal of the National Cancer Institute* 92 (2000): 128–135.

Vitaliano, P. P.; Scanlan, J. M.; Ochs, H. D.; Syrjala, K.; Siegler, I.; and Snyder, E. A. "Psychosocial Stress Moderates the Relationship of Cancer History with Natural Killer Cell Activity." *Annals of Behavioral Medicine* 20 (1998): 199–208.

Wandi, S.; Gandhi, R.; and Snedeker, S. "Critical Evaluation of Heptachlor and Heptachlor Epoxide's Breast Cancer Risk Pesticide." 1998. www.cfe.Cornell.Edu/bcerf/CriticalEval/Pesticide/CE.heptachlor.pdf

Whittemore, A.S.; Wu-Williams, A. H.; Lee, M.; et al. "Diet, Physical Activity, and Colorectal Cancer among Chinese in North America and China." *Journal of the National Cancer Institute* 82 (1990): 915–926.

World Cancer Research Fund and the American Institute of Cancer Research. *Food, Nutrition, and the Prevention of Cancer: A Global Perspective.* Washington, D.C.: American Institute of Cancer Research, 1997.

Index

Note: An Index of Recipe Titles can be found on pages ix–x.